The HEART
of a
Woman

How to look after the heart you
give to the world.

by

Gill Barham

The Heart of a Woman
How to look after the heart you give to the world - Gill Barham
pg. 1

The HEART of a Woman

How to look after the heart you give to the world.

Gill Barham
Copyright © Gill Barham
Date first Published: 17th November 2016, London, England

All Rights Reserved

Published by RADIO W.O.R.K.S. WORLD

The Heart of a Woman
How to look after the heart you give to the world - Gill Barham
pg. 2

I would like to dedicate this book firstly to my lovely family.

To my husband and partner of 34 years, Peter who is still my very best friend in the whole world, who gives me the space to "do my thing" and is the best father that I've ever known.

Also to my son Matt who allowed me to use his personal story (eventually) and who I am very proud of.

To my youngest daughter Lydia, who designed the book cover, and who shows the world how to have the best time, has the brightest smile and the most generous of natures.

And to my eldest daughter Ellie, who supplied some of the illustrations; is beautiful and talented and has found a way to be herself in the world as a feminine but powerful young woman.

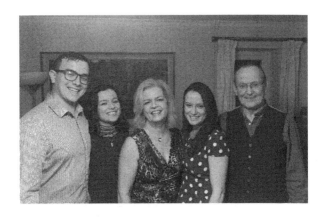

The Heart of a Woman
How to look after the heart you give to the world - Gill Barham

I would also like to recognise and acknowledge the help, support and inspiration from the women who are my friends and mentors, without whom this book would never have been written: my good friend and Pilates teacher Sarah Andrews, the "wind beneath my wings" Marina Nani, my "Golden Muse" Chrisoula Sirigou and the incomparable duo that is Marion Bevington and Cheryl Chapman. A big thank you too, to the lovely Anne Davison for her proof reading skills

Oh and by the way, I have spent many happy hours writing the chapters of this book on the train, in local café's, but more often in the chair of Paul Watts Hairdressing Salon (a true young entrepreneur who will go far).

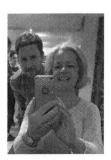

Thank you to all who believed that I have a book inside me. Now dear lady, it's your turn. Because if I can do it, so can you.

The Heart of a Woman
How to look after the heart you give to the world - Gill Barham
pg. 4

CONTENTS

PREFACE

PROLOGUE

The Heart of a Woman
How to look after the heart you give to the world - Gill Barham

Foreword

This is a must-read publication by Gill Barham, Lifestyle Coach. This book serves as a reference compendium relating to issues that matter to the wellbeing of women, yet, having said that, men are not excluded. I would have loved to have this publication in the early 1980's when I was a health education officer.

The book starts off with light bulb moments and with the insight that *we make a living by what we get, but we make a life by what we give* and the book flows beautifully into revealing the heart that you give to the world; with the reminder of your Divine Essence then the book beautifully illustrates the profound reality that *the most reliable way to predict your future is to create it.*

In reading, you are skilfully guided through the 5Ps for a **Healthy Starter Programme**™ inclusive of how to maintain a healthy cardio-vascular system and a healthy body with a range of nutrients.

Do you understand your Total Body Blueprint™? Read this book for more insight.

The book gently guides you to understand and to know that good health is all about creating good habits and that the legacy that you create is the legacy that you leave.

There is much to gain from this book for people within a wide age range. You are taken through discourse, research, knowledge and facts to the conclusion that wellbeing is fundamental to your overall health and that wellbeing enables you to successfully overcome difficulties and more importantly focus on your purpose in life.

The Heart of a Woman
How to look after the heart you give to the world - Gill Barham
pg. 6

Well-being is crucial to a healthy life and it is a fine balance between relationships with yourself and others, having a nutritious and life sustaining diet, getting enough exercise, maintain healthy cardio-vascular and immune systems as well as sustaining a positive outlook on life.

I highly recommend Gill's book that is easy to read with nuggets of wisdom.

Dr Neslyn Watson-Druée, CBE FCGI FRCN

Author of Fly High Land Safely: The Definitive Book on Career Transition for Executives. The Beacon Technique Leadership: From Impossible to Possible and The Beacon leadership Technique: The Book on Building Effective Relationships for High Flying Executives

About the Author

When I first met Gill I knew I liked her straight away, at first I thought it was the familiarity of her likeness to Marilyn Monroe with her blonde hair and big smile, but now I know it was something more.

As I began to find out more about her, I recognised that it was her "bedside manner", clearly kept from her time as a nurse, that was so endearing.

When Gill became a mentee of mine I realised that not only did she care for people, and I mean really care, but I could also see that she had the knowledge to be able to help them in all aspects of their lives.

The Heart of a Woman
How to look after the heart you give to the world - Gill Barham
pg. 7

Her passion and drive are infectious and it has been a delight to be a part of her development in being able to get her message out to many others. In fact, her 'mission' to help 1,000,000 others!

I can see that Gill is living on purpose and she has found her WHY!

Gill also reminded me that as a busy woman I had to look after myself if I wanted to be healthy enough to help others in my business (I help others to Find Your WHY!). She was right and so I made the decision to improve my health.

I was thrilled to be a part of her on-line programme, which I could follow despite being an International Jet Setting Speaker with little routine and very rarely home. The programme was exactly what I was looking for.

Gill's ability to teach and have tangible steps for me to follow made it possible to change my future health with both success and ease and the bonus was that it was convenient to follow anywhere in the world.

It is because of my personal health achievements from working with Gill that I can, without hesitation, say that if you are looking for a guide to living the healthy, happy and fulfilled lifestyle you want, then this is the book for you.

Cheryl Chapman

Creator of The Find Your WHY! Foundation

The Heart of a Woman
How to look after the heart you give to the world - Gill Barham

Preface

This book is based on the principles of Wellbeing. There are a variety of definitions, but all with the same core values:

This is WHO's definition as contained in its constitution: *"Health is a state of complete physical, mental and social well-being and not merely the absence of disease or infirmity."*

Anthony Robbins sums up wellbeing in terms of The 6 Human Needs:
1. certainty
2. variety
3. significance
4. contribution
5. love and connection
6. personal growth

"Wellbeing and abundance are directly related to the amount of attention you place on self-care, self-growth and self-improvement." Tony Robbins

and this is a quote from New Economics Foundation -
"Because of this dynamic nature, high levels of wellbeing mean that we are more-able to respond to difficult circumstances, to innovate and constructively engage with other people and the world around us...... there is also a strong case for regarding well-being as an ultimate goal of human endeavour."

And finally, a dictionary definition: *"Wellbeing is enjoying a contented state of good health, happiness and prosperity"*
The Heart of a Woman
How to look after the heart you give to the world - Gill Barham

So here is my question…. How important is it to you to be happy, healthy and prosperous? To have a sense of wellbeing?

Perhaps you are here reading this book because you are feeling a bit low in spirits or lacking in energy?

Possibly you have some health concerns, or there are some annoying symptoms starting to show up, and:

If you are a man:
a) you are almost certainly ignoring the signs and
b) what are you doing reading this book? (joking – please read on, you will learn a lot and don't forget to share with your favourite women)

or

c) If you are a woman you are too busy looking after everything and everyone else to do anything about it.

(Well perhaps that's not you but someone you know, right?)

Maybe you are reading this book because your work life balance is out of whack and you're looking for some other way to "be" in the world.

And it may even be that outwardly you are putting on a brave face but inwardly you feel confused, run down, perhaps frustrated or even afraid for your physical and financial future?

The Heart of a Woman
How to look after the heart you give to the world - Gill Barham
pg. 10

Well imagine a life instead where every day is easy, where every day is exciting and rewarding and you are SO on top of your health that you feel energised and capable of enjoying what lies ahead, both in the short term and the long term.

You are looking forward to a future where you can be with the people you want, wherever you want, doing what you want.

You are financially free, or at least on your way to securing a more stable and abundant future.

You are thinking, saying and BEING the true you and you feel fulfilled and respected and know that you are going to be able to leave an amazing legacy.

Does that sound like a great way to live? Would you want to know how to achieve this? Then read on lovely lady, because I am here to talk to you about your Heart - both the heart that is in your body and the one you give to the world. I am going to give you easy to follow, proven solutions for how you can heal your heart and change your life. I hope that you are inspired by my book and would ask that you share it with any woman that is dear to you.

Love Gill

Gill Barham

But before we begin there is something I think you should know....

The Heart of a Woman
How to look after the heart you give to the world - Gill Barham
pg. 11

Prologue

It's November 2012, and if you were with me you would be sitting opposite a petite, grey haired lady with her glasses on a beaded string around her neck, wearing a dark blue nurses uniform; she has a soft welsh accent.

"Well Gill, I have your results, you have protein in your sample so there is likely to be an infection, your blood results aren't good, your cholesterol is high I'm afraid and your blood pressure is too, actually really high for you, I've never seen this in the 20 years I've known you, and you are quite a few kilos heavier than last time you were here. You are not looking yourself. What's going on?"

"Ugh well I'm not surprised Dawn I feel dreadful, really low, I'm not sleeping, my hormones are all out of whack and I have no energy or interest in doing anything really. I have had the most stressful summer, my elderly father is becoming more dependant, I'm worried about my youngest daughter who has struggled a bit with her first A level year, and of course work doesn't get any easier; it's all got too much I think."

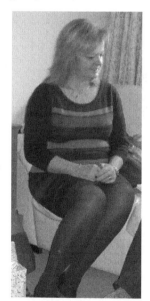

Me, not looking or feeling great at all

The Heart of a Woman
How to look after the heart you give to the world - Gill Barham
pg. 12

"OK, there are some things we can do; obviously, you'll need a course of antibiotics, and I can make you an appointment with the GP to look at what you need to take to lower your BP and cholesterol and she will discuss with you maybe about having some antidepressants or some counselling perhaps? Tell me are you feeling like you want to harm yourself? "

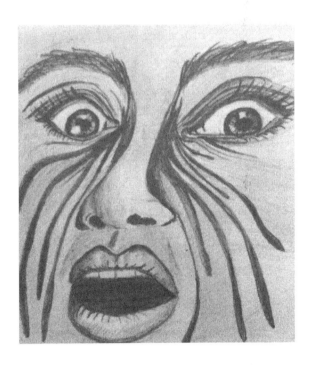

The Heart of a Woman
How to look after the heart you give to the world - Gill Barham

CHAPTER I

The Light Bulb Moment

Have you heard the expression, hindsight is a wonderful thing?

Do you remember the question that Dawn asked of me?

"Tell me are you feeling like you want to harm yourself?"

"Whaaaaat? No... do I seem that bad? This can't be right. this is like a repeat of what happened with my mum, I have always been told that I am just like my mum... by my age she was depressed, overweight and had high blood pressure and cholesterol too. I can't go down this route, this is really scary. Look Dawn, as you know I hate the thought of taking statins or anti-depressants, I know too much about the side effects. I'll take the antibiotics but I will find other ways to deal with the rest."

So over that next week you'll find me taking a look at why I was where I was, weighing up the pros and cons – looking at what I loved about my life, and what wasn't so good. It became abundantly clear that the main source of stress was my job, well, actually, not the job but specifically the person who was my boss. For the previous five years I was employed by a National Federation of Sport and I worked as part of a small team for the woman we all called "Miss Management" – a cross between JK Rowling and Jekyll and Hyde. For the past two years I had found working for her almost

The Heart of a Woman
How to look after the heart you give to the world - Gill Barham
pg. 14

impossible but kept my "part time" job on – working more and more hours with no recognition, no job security and no support.

Is this a familiar scenario to you? Being paid for a part-time job but working full time hours? Have you had others take the credit for your work?

I had known for some time that she was not good for me. I recognised that I had allowed her to affect my mental and physical health, my relationships, my confidence, my spirit and get into my heart. It had been such a gradual downwards spiral, that I hadn't realised how bad things had become.

Has that ever happened to you or someone you know? It helps when you can see things in a different light doesn't it? ….. when you look back "in hindsight."

So I resigned from the job that week and booked to have lunch with my friend, Pilates teacher and health coach Sarah. We are about the same age, and in contrast, she looked amazing, slim, glowing in health, happy and fulfilled.

"Well, Gill it's about time!! That woman has a lot to answer for. Why don't you come and join our health team, you'd be great with your nursing background and I think you'd make a fab Pilates teacher; you know so much already after 11 years working with me! You would learn so much about how to help your son too".

You see the "straw that broke the camel's back"; the event that tipped me over into illness that I could no longer ignore, happened just a few months before.

The Heart of a Woman
How to look after the heart you give to the world - Gill Barham
pg. 15

Only moments from death.

On this day in July 2012 if you were with me we are sitting in a bland, white room, the only sound is of distant phones ringing, we can smell disinfectant and sense fear and sadness in the air. In walks a short, young man with a dark straggly beard, a stethoscope around his neck and a white coat.

Despite his Asian appearance, his accent is Scottish. *"Mrs. Barham, we have got to the bottom of your son's condition. I know he has spent nearly 3 weeks at your GP and various visits to the hospital, so it must have been very worrying for you. Matthew has epiglottitis; this is where the flap at the top of the wind pipe becomes inflamed and swollen and can block the passage of air. It is normally seen in the very elderly or in young babies, so it is very rare to see this in a 20-year-old, fit looking guy like Matthew. We have him on the right medication now, so hopefully he will be home in a few days."*

I remember the feeling of relief for us both, as we had finally got a diagnosis after so many days of worry and extreme levels of pain for Matt. So I went home, and did when any normal person would do... I looked the condition up on Google! (other search engines are available).

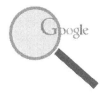

The Heart of a Woman
How to look after the heart you give to the world - Gill Barham

BUT....this just made me feel worse! You see Epiglottitis is a life-threatening condition, and in that moment I recall the hairs standing up on the back of my neck as I remembered the car journey only two days before where I was thinking to myself, *"I wonder if I should have called an ambulance, I'm not sure I'm going to get him there in time his breathing is getting worse.. I wonder if I can remember how to do a tracheotomy"*

Have you ever felt helpless and unsure about what to do for someone you love?

Well, Matt did recover slowly, but within a week of returning to University in October, he developed tonsillitis, a regular occurrence all through his teenage years. So although he was "fixed", we were still not getting to the route of his life-threatening episode.

So I knew in my heart that the story couldn't end there.

Using a plaster to fix a disaster

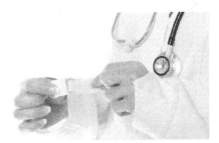

Back to November, and this time imagine we are sitting in a meeting room in a hotel. It has oak panels on the walls, low lighting and there is a petite woman with short dark hair standing in front of a

The Heart of a Woman
How to look after the heart you give to the world - Gill Barham
pg. 17

projector screen. *"So I think we have all seen and understood this evening that the root of illness is inflammation and that in order to achieve optimum health, we need a healthy gut, but more essentially, a strong heart, one that is emotionally and physiologically nurtured."*

In that moment it was clear that my path from that day was to learn how to do just that, for myself, for my son and for anyone whose life I touched. As I started my own journey back to being well, and to being able to help hundreds of others achieve wellbeing, my first lesson was in the importance of the gut to good health. During the trauma of that summer I had a sense that Matt's IBS (Irritable Bowel Syndrome) had a significant role to play in his illness but there was not one medical professional that seemed interested in my view when he was being treated. You see we were in the ENT – Ear Nose and Throat Department, not the Gastroenterology Department.

So I was first in the queue to speak to the naturopath and nutritionist that evening. "So you are saying that if a gut isn't working well, then this can affect all parts of the body, even your moods and lower your immune system?"

"Yes and your son would have been particularly vulnerable as he had just suffered a few months of flare up of his IBS, but there are ways to heal the gut and improve his overall health."

Looks can be deceiving.

It wasn't until I started to study nutrition and health that I really began to grow my understanding of the fundamentals of natural healing. As a student nurse, we had no training in nutrition, (you

The Heart of a Woman
How to look after the heart you give to the world - Gill Barham
pg. 18

may not be aware that our bright and brilliant student doctors get minimal information on nutrition as part of their 5-year training). I have always been interested in complimentary, preventative and holistic therapies, and in more recent years my research and study has helped me to focus on the real route to optimum health. I believe now that there are indeed two key systems that define our emotional and physical wellness: the GUT and the HEART.

What is clear, is that we can never tell how healthy a person is by outwardly appearances. You may have experienced first or second hand the sudden death of person and been shocked as they "looked" healthy, young, slim and fit even?

Gut reaction.

Through the trauma of Matt's illness; I recall my feelings of helplessness as he was pushed from doctors' surgeries to emergency rooms and hospital wards. All along, my instincts were telling me that he was in real trouble, and I believe that every mother knows her child better than anyone else does. **I want to encourage you as a woman to trust your instincts, believe in yourself and listen to your gut reactions about your life and those you care about.** I also understand that this has to start with self-care and self-awareness.

If like me, you are putting everyone else first, perhaps taking a back seat with your health when you know you are the rudder of your ship, then I want to empower you to take some action today so that you don't become vulnerable. I also want to inspire you to learn some basic principles of how to live a life of wellness and to help those around you whom you love to avoid my fate.

The Heart of a Woman
How to look after the heart you give to the world - Gill Barham
pg. 19

"In Life You Can Either be a Good Example, or a Horrible Warning"

Catherine Aird

The Heart of a Woman
How to look after the heart you give to the world - Gill Barham
pg. 20

You see, what I didn't tell you is that I lost my mum to a Pulmonary Embolus, a cardiovascular-related accident, when I was twenty eight and thirty weeks pregnant with my first child. She was only fifty six years old. She had suffered many years of unhappiness and stress in her marriage with my father who was controlling at times; the life and soul of the party in company but miserable at home. So, next year at the time of writing…. I will be fifty six. I have no intention of being the "horrible warning"; leaving my beautiful, talented and loving children without a mum, and a grandma who will love and cherish their future offspring.

So here I am, four years on, helping other women to look after their hearts, like I am striving to look after mine; taking care of my physical and emotional needs, learning to cope with the curve balls that we all experience in life. My own personal development has led me to the "heart" of the matter:

- To find a way to earn money, and let's face it we all need to do that, that better suits my passion.
- To work with like-minded souls with the same integrity and commitment.
- To fulfill my true purpose and leave a legacy for my family, and to the world.
- To understand the over-riding root of illness and disease and how to offer simple, proven solutions to women just like you to live happier, healthier and more prosperous lives.
- To boldly go where… (oops got carried away there with the Star Trek reference!!)

And my mission is:

To build a team to save 1 million lives a year, every year.

The Heart of a Woman
How to look after the heart you give to the world - Gill Barham
pg. 21

"We make a living by what we get, but we make a life by what we give."
Winston Churchill

CHAPTER II

The Heart Within

Heart disease, or more accurately, cardiovascular disease is the biggest killer in the western world. Yearly deaths account for as many lives as the next seven causes of death combined.

Despite big pharma and medical science providing health professionals with an array of heart disease medications; surgeries and interventions to address high blood pressure, cholesterol levels, angina, peripheral vascular disease, and associated conditions, heart disease is still on the rise.

So you may be thinking, why is this?

Have you noticed that we are seeing more people who are overweight? Obesity is on the rise with 1 in 3 adults and shockingly, 1 in 4 of our 11-16 year olds in the UK classed as clinically obese. Type 2 diabetes has doubled in the last 10 years and is set to rise unless we address the causes now. Autoimmune diseases, such as fibromyalgia, ME, and Rheumatoid Arthritis are also on the increase and we are witnessing more chronic illness and memory disorders.

I believe our 21st century living is to blame – the major disease mega trends are mostly due to lifestyle choices.

The Heart of a Woman
How to look after the heart you give to the world - Gill Barham
pg. 23

Have you also noticed that we are living in a world of convenience, fast food, quick fix health care, overwhelm and imbalance? Even if you think you are taking good care of yourself, our 21st century world is making it very difficult for us to be healthy and happy. In this book we look at why this is and what we can do about it.

Big is Best

I recall that 13 years ago we went as a family to Florida in the USA for the first time. On arrival, looking around the house we had rented for our stay, I was struck by how big the rooms were, I was amazed by the size of the washing machine, the fridge, the spacious, imposing cars and trucks, the size of the roads, the diners, the plates of food and the size of the people!!!

Like me you may have witnessed that in Europe and especially the UK, we tend to follow US trends, and over the years since that trip, I have witnessed, guess what? American style fridges, big trucks and 4x4 cars, widening motorways, bigger portions, and yes, bigger people.

The influence of the western lifestyle is reaching across the globe and so heart disease is becoming a GLOBAL HEALTH PROBLEM.

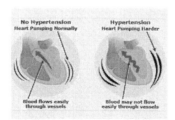

The Heart of a Woman
How to look after the heart you give to the world - Gill Barham

The heart you give to the world

Now this book is mostly aimed at you if you are a woman, but guys, you can read on, because I am certain you have at least one important woman in your life who needs this information.
Our culture has changed over the past thirty years. Couples are starting their families later, and often running into problems conceiving.

There are now more new mothers over the age of 40 than under 20; a phenomenon last seen after the Second World War.

Stay-at–home mums (or dads) are often viewed with derision; although thankfully there are many more opportunities to work from home these days that give care givers the fulfilment and freedom of choice (more on that later). Also, although a major benefit in many ways, the Information Technology (IT) era has changed our home lives. We are constantly connected and "on" all the time. The profile of a typical family unit has changed and we are more likely to be living a good distance away from our relatives than close by. I see that there is more pressure on younger women to be working, raising a family, earning enough to get a house, a bigger house, a newer car, better holidays, or perhaps to pay school fees, or more significantly, even just to keep paying the bills.

When is there any time for fun? For nourishment, for peace, for exercise for self-care?

Is this the legacy we want to leave behind for our daughters, nieces, grand-daughters, god daughters? Can we find a better way to be fulfilled, valued and live a healthy and happy life too?

The Heart of a Woman
How to look after the heart you give to the world - Gill Barham
pg. 25

"We are all born with a divine essence, it's for you to develop that essence into greatness. Don't ignore your inner greatness and take your dream to an early grave."
Marina Nani

The Heart of a Woman
How to look after the heart you give to the world - Gill Barham

Do you remember what you wanted from life when you were 10? 20? 30? How does that dream compare to your life path now?

Now, I do respect that as a woman it is a valuable thing to have choice in our lives, but I believe that some women increasingly feel pressure to prove themselves; to compete with men, and this is damaging the "heart of a woman". This has been going on for a few decades.

I listened recently to Inga Beale being interviewed by Kirsty Young on one of our great traditional British radio shows, Desert Island Discs. As a senior executive in the Insurance industry in the 1980's, Inga talked about the way in which she modified her behaviour to "fit- in" with the male culture. (She was the only female in a team of 35 male underwriters.) She would go to the pub after work, took up rugby and gained a reputation for being tough. She eventually worked out that this was not serving her and that she needed to escape from the very aggressive and chauvinist world she found herself in. After running away to tour the world, she discovered a woman boss who had found a way to be effective, **and** feminine. She under-took self-confidence courses and personal development workshops and found her own way to be authentic in the environment in which she worked.

Back in the days when I last worked for someone else, not that long ago, this really hadn't changed very much. My CEO was the "army type" who always picked the only guy on our team to talk to or consult with, on projects. Perhaps you feel undervalued too?

The result of living and working in a way that doesn't resonate with you can be very stressful.

The Heart of a Woman
How to look after the heart you give to the world - Gill Barham
pg. 27

Cardiovascular diseases accounts for more deaths in the western world than any other disease by far. For example, 1 in 2.4 women die of heart disease, whereas 1 in 30 women die of breast cancer. (Yet it is breast cancer that we focus on and hear most about, would you agree?) My research shows that more women are actually more worried about dementia than heart disease too. This seems to be because there are perceived remedies for cancer and heart disease, but not from Alzheimer's or Dementia.

Isn't it just men that die of heart attacks?

No, definitely not. In the USA there is some form of coronary event every 29 seconds, a person dies of a heart attack every 1 minute and 53% of these are WOMEN. Only 7 out of 10 women survive their first heart attack.

There are currently 3.5 million women in the UK living with cardiovascular disease and the British Heart Foundation predicts that rates are set to rise.

You are what you eat.

When I trained as a nurse in the 90's we had very little information relatively speaking to today about how lifestyle choices affect us. We were still smoking, even our GPs smoked; we were encouraged to eat low fat food, eat ready meals, count calories to lose weight, and choose diet/no sugar drinks. We know now that much of this information was ill-formed, badly-researched and reported. For example, the LOW FAT revolution came about largely due to the research of Ancel Keys in the 1960's who studied 21 countries to see if the reduction in high fat foods would improve cardiovascular

The Heart of a Woman
How to look after the heart you give to the world - Gill Barham
pg. 28

health. His conclusions were that we should indeed adopt a LOW FAT diet based on his results, but it has since been highlighted that these were manipulated to achieve his theory. He selected only the seven nations that proved his hypothesis, and in fact subsequent information would suggest that the results were more likely to be because of the simultaneous reduction in the consumption of sugar during the study.

I am happy to say that this bears no comparison to the increasing advances in scientific knowledge and awareness of metabolic processes today around the role that lifestyle choices play in our long-term health. I am fortunate to be associated with eminent scientists, PhDs, medical professionals, nutritional and herbal experts who are dedicated to the cause of the prevention and reversal of disease, and in particular cardiovascular disease and the microbiome: the impact of gut flora on health.

> **How much more would we gain by concentrating on** *wellness awareness* **over** *cancer awareness***?**

www.theLifestyleLeader.co.uk

The Heart of a Woman
How to look after the heart you give to the world - Gill Barham
pg. 29

It is my belief that there has never been a better time to *learn more* and *do more* to protect yourself.

This book will help you to look at this in more detail.

The wellness industry is the biggest in the world, it survived the recent recession because we all now want to look and feel younger, live longer and stay in good health.

It's too noisy for me.

Would you agree with me that we have so much access now to information on health issues, that it's very common to be overwhelmed by all the opinions and facts that we have at our fingertips? You may even be your own GP (Google Practitioner) like me!

Sometimes this works out all for the good.

James Le Fann – health reporter at the UKs Daily Telegraph published a recent post on how a British woman did her own research on the fact that PPI (Proton Pump Inhibitors) drugs such as Omeprazole, may produce side effects such as muscle weakness and fatigue. Quick version: the medical profession was stumped by her symptoms, so she was empowered in this instance to take action by the research she undertook on the internet, and stopped taking her medications. Her symptoms went away.

The Heart of a Woman
How to look after the heart you give to the world - Gill Barham
pg. 30

But sometimes your browsing may lead to nightmares!!

Have you ever looked at your symptoms online and diagnosed yourself with an array of diseases? Or frightened yourself by imagining the worst? "Yep, it's definitely early onset senile dementia", or "I must have a sluggish thyroid", "Ahhh I think it must be legionnaires disease" or even "When was the last incidence of the plague??"

So would it be fair to say that you may need some help? Well that is my intention: to educate, to make things simple, to take away the fear and provide you with natural solutions and alternatives – so that you can choose a life of wellbeing.

Why is now a good time to take control of your health? Because in the UK the NHS is overwhelmed - 1 million people are seen every 36 hours.

Life expectancy is rising (the average age of a woman is now 82 years) - but so is chronic illness. **The average age of living without disease and in full health in the UK is only 58.**

Here is what I believe:
Stress, whether perceived or unperceived, is a major factor in early death from cardiovascular disease and our lifestyle choices play a significant factor in your risk.

The Heart of a Woman
How to look after the heart you give to the world - Gill Barham
pg. 31

"The most reliable way to predict your future is to create it."
Abraham Lincoln

CHAPTER III

What's Your Poison?

Our 21st century, high octane, multi- tasking, busy, busy lifestyles may be commonplace, but is it healthy?
You may not have noticed that the way you live is having an impact on your health. Whether it is just a few aches and pains, lack of energy, infertility/hormonal problems, peri-menopausal/post-menopausal symptoms, repeated colds or infections, IBS, weight gain, migraines, fatigue, or more serious issues, you might like to take a step back for a minute to check yourself out!

A GREAT place to start is to look, and I mean REALLY LOOK, at what habits or situations there are in your life that have been happening gradually over the last few years that you have become to accept as normal, even if they are undesirable or uncomfortable?

Quick Start Heart Check
Place a tick on any and all that are relevant for you today.

Increase in stress levels ☐
Weight gain (or unexplained weight loss) ☐
Too much time spent on social media ☐
Lack of exercise/fresh air ☐
Working long hours ☐

The Heart of a Woman
How to look after the heart you give to the world - Gill Barham
pg. 33

Long commutes to work ☐
Carrying on through illness ☐
Spending less time with family and/or friends ☐
Eating "on the go" ☐
Reliance on convenience foods (including your lunch time "healthy" salad from Pret or M&S) ☐
The daily glass of wine/beer to unwind... Which may turn into 2 or more! ☐
Putting everyone else first (yes, I'm talking to you!) ☐
Being too busy for hobbies or "me time" ☐
Not taking breaks or holidays ☐
Trying to be perfect or do it all ☐

Tot up your score:
under 5 – how can you get it to 3?
Under 10 – you are pushing too hard
Over 10 – wow, your heart is at real risk.

GET DOWN AND DIRTY
In the longer term you might take a look at your daily/weekly/monthly routines.
Perhaps you could keep a diary for a month or two?
Chart:

- What you eat
- Where you eat
- What you are drinking, (include caffeine, alcohol, sweet stuff)
- How much sleep you are getting

The Heart of a Woman
How to look after the heart you give to the world - Gill Barham
pg. 34

Plus, how many hours spent:

- Working
- Working at home after work hours
- On social media
- With friends/family
- Exercising
- Outside
- On daily chores
- On hobbies
- Alone/quiet time
- Commuting
- Rushing around with the kids – school, after school clubs, hobbies, friends etc.

By now, you should have a picture of where your focus is...

So, I would ask you….
Are you getting the balance right for you?
Is it nourishing you? Both in mind and body….
Is it nourishing your relationships?
Is it keeping you fit and healthy?
Are you setting a good example for those around you?
Is it sustainable?

If the answer is YES, then that's AWESOME! FANTASTIC!

But if it's a NO... Then how can you start to redress the balance?

The Heart of a Woman
How to look after the heart you give to the world - Gill Barham
pg. 35

In this book I will suggest some small steps to change the things you want to change. It is however, vital that you work on the BIG PICTURE of what you want to achieve FIRST. **I will help you to do just that in more detail in chapter VIII.**

The Perfect Day

In the meantime, you may like to take some time to sit alone, with no distractions, close your eyes and imagine what your perfect day would look like.

- Who are you laughing with?
- Where are you?
- What are you eating?
- Who are you working alongside?
- What nice things do you own?
- What are you wearing?
- Where are you planning to holiday?
- For how long?
- Who are you helping?
- What are you looking forward to?

If you can re visit this VISION of your perfect day, EVERY day, then you will find that your actions will be more aligned with your values and dreams... and ultimately,

This will drive you towards a happier, healthier, wealthier and more fulfilled future: Having a true sense of Wellbeing.

Now... How do I know this...?

Is it because I have it sorted? Nooooooooo! Definitely not!

The Heart of a Woman
How to look after the heart you give to the world - Gill Barham
pg. 36

I am still a work in progress, you know my story. I know how it feels to be so passionate about something (e.g. money, a job, a career, a business, study) or somebody, (e.g. children, partner, parents, friends or a cause) where it drives you to keep going! Even when you know you are running out of steam and you know you are in denial about it!

But here's what I've found... Sometimes taking the time to re-evaluate what's important, and listen to what those around you are saying to you, (Why are you still working? Come and sit down for a while, the chores will wait til tomorrow, you never switch off, we never spend any time together, etc.) Is the BEST investment of your time EVER. I believe that:

"Practicing a healthy lifestyle, may make for a perfect life."

www.theLifestyleLeader.co.uk

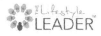

The Heart of a Woman
How to look after the heart you give to the world - Gill Barham

Then you will be more able to take the necessary ACTION to tweak and re-organise where you can. And because I have made loads of mistakes myself long the way, I have used my experience to create The **Your H.E.A.R.T. Matters™** Programme.

This is a 5 step blueprint for a Healthier, Wealthier and Happier you, based on years of self-development, working with mentors, studying the fundamentals of functional nutrition and writing, blogging, teaching and speaking about natural health and lifestyle solutions.

Why is this important?

You are the rudder of your ship! You need to take care of yourself first so that you can take care of the other people in your life who are important to you.

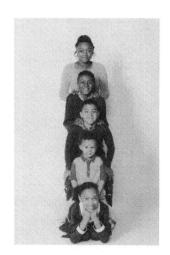

Like the oxygen mask warning on your flight – "please secure your own mask in place first before helping others".

The Heart of a Woman
How to look after the heart you give to the world - Gill Barham
pg. 38

The 5 P's

1

When I work with my clients we kick off with **The Healthy Starter Programme™.** This does exactly what it says on the tin. Here I help them to understand the likely physical and emotional stresses of our 21st Century living that may be affecting them. My clients learn how to purify, fortify and protect their bodies and get started on the path to Elite Health. When you understand the factors that are affecting your weight, your concentration and brain power, your stamina, your hormonal health and your risk of disease, you will be able to create a better sense of control over your health for the future. This will allow you to be able to have more certainty for your future by knowing more about how to **PREPARE** for that desired sense of wellbeing.

2

If you are dedicated to pharmaceuticals and popping pills, then the next module will be something quite new to you. My clients learn the 3 easy, natural steps they need to take every day to nourish their bodies. With **The Essential Energy Elevator™** you will learn how to **PREVENT** illness and disease, how to combat the complications of common disorders and how to increase and optimise the way your body functions every day. Wellness is all about creating good habits by making small changes that you can maintain, and this module helps you to do just that.

The Heart of a Woman
How to look after the heart you give to the world - Gill Barham
pg. 39

3

One of my major passions is to give my clients a tangible way; a proven roadmap for achieving financial security to **PROSPER**. I created **The Advanced S.U.C.C.E.S.S. Solution™** to show that there is a way of generating an income other than the conventional exchanging time for money model, without having to invest serious time or money. My clients learn how they can use their skills, or learn some new ones, whilst working towards their own financial success rather than on behalf of someone else. When you have a method of creating an income that fits in with your family and lifestyle commitments, when you earn money while you sleep and when you can develop flexibility in your work life, then you will know true wellbeing and enjoy a sense of fulfilment as you work to leave a legacy. At the very least, my clients are able to pay for the higher quality food and nutrition, making better choices to achieve Elite Health.

4

I also help my clients discover the best way to achieve their very own version of success and **PURPOSE** in their lives with **The Rapid Realignment Process™** We take a good honest look at what they love and what they don't love about their current life. When you undertake this process you can develop a road map for success. It's a bit like starting any journey, if you put Liverpool into your satnav, but not the starting co-ordinates, what chance will you have of reaching your destination? This exercise is so important for all aspects of wellbeing and covers the 6 human needs, the 8 areas of lifestyle that I look at personally on a regular basis so that I can steer my own ship or navigate my way safely to my desired destination, albeit not necessarily in a straight line!

The Heart of a Woman
How to look after the heart you give to the world - Gill Barham
pg. 40

5

Once we have some basic principles of health covered then the next step is to refine these for my clients on an individual basis. **The Total Body Blueprint™** is all about looking a little deeper into the individual body systems to support their journey to wellness. When you know what your strengths and weaknesses are, you have much more opportunity to achieve better health and maintain it. I will help you to balance and rebuild where necessary, to **PERFECT** your regime and to sustain and support for longevity.

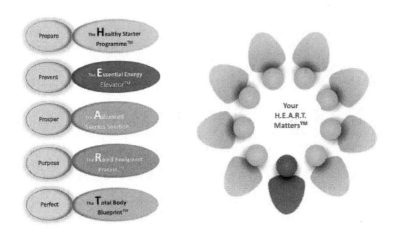

So are you ready *to explore the 5 P's in more detail?*

The Heart of a Woman
How to look after the heart you give to the world - Gill Barham
pg. 41

CHAPTER IV

"What is the world's most expensive bed? The hospital bed."
Steve Jobs

Prepare

We will dig deep in this chapter into the three areas that you need to understand in order to develop a way to counteract the effects of our modern-day lifestyles.

Unless you have a sense of what is making it difficult for you to lose weight, have more energy, stop your aches and pains, think more clearly and feel like you did in your teens and twenties, then it is more likely that you will succumb to ill health and worry about what will happen as you age.

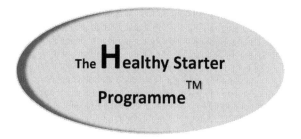

The **H**ealthy Starter Programme™

The Heart of a Woman
How to look after the heart you give to the world - Gill Barham
pg. 42

IV.1 CHEMICAL OVERLOAD

I believe that there are many health issues which are the result of two very interconnected problems. One is Nutritional Deficiencies, which I will cover in a later chapter but it is chemical overload that we're going to talk about first.

Are YOU a toxic waste dump?

Our bodies were not designed to live in our 21st century very toxic world. There are 2 types of toxins that we are going to cover that are chemically overloading our very delicate systems: exogenous and endogenous toxins.

So, let's look first at the **exogenous toxins**. The ones from outside the body.

We are all exposed to pollution on a daily basis, whether you live in the countryside, the city or the town. Well known pollutants such as fumes from industry, cigarette smoke, car fumes, or farming sprays are everyday hazards, but it is also the pollutants that are in and around your environment, your house or your office space, that build the toxic levels in your body too. Such as:
- freshly scented candles
- household/ office cleaners
- room sprays

We know that processed foods are not good for us, e.g. foods such as takeaways, pastries, ready meals, packaged food etc. that are

The Heart of a Woman
How to look after the heart you give to the world - Gill Barham
pg. 43

high in sugars, chemicals and bad fats but you may not be aware that even our healthier foods are often treated with chemicals to preserve shelf life and appeal.

I bought a salad from a well-known high street "healthy choice" food outlet recently, but there were 25 ingredients just in that salad, and the majority were not food items that I recognised.

POP goes the weasel.

These chemical toxins are known as POPs or Persistent Organic Pollutants. Chemicals such as herbicides and pesticides, preservatives and enzymes that are used in our food so that it can be stored for up to six months or a year at a time. We also have chemicals in our water, e.g:
- the volatile organics washed into the rivers from the land
- chlorine
- fluoride
- heavy metals

These levels vary depending on where your water supply comes from but they will be acting like chemical toxins too. Our individual reactions will all vary to these POPs.

Other environmental toxins we need to be aware of, are in our personal care products. **The average woman uses 300 chemicals on her skin every day** depending on which ranges of hair, skin and makeup products she uses.

The Heart of a Woman
How to look after the heart you give to the world - Gill Barham
pg. 44

The over-exposure to the common chemical BPA sets us more at risk of cancer. This is present in our drinking water bottles (especially when they are at room temperature or above) and BPA is used as a coating on till receipts to stop the ink from smudging. (I never accept a til receipt unless I need it)
We also experience toxicity through:

- Mercury fillings
- Electromagnetic toxins – iPhones, smartphones, iPads, laptops etc.

Oops - Female overload!!

One less known or talked about toxins is Xenoestrogens. These are "false" oestrogens that act like the hormone oestrogen and produce hormonal imbalances in our bodies. This causes conditions like endometriosis, PCOS, PMS, increased menopausal symptoms and infertility. **It is estimated that one in eight couples in the UK is infertile** and you'll see from this graph that 25% of the infertility is actually "unexplained".

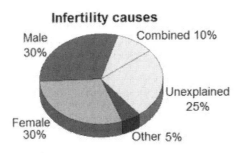

The Heart of a Woman
How to look after the heart you give to the world - Gill Barham

These high levels of Xenoestrogens are affecting our men too in terms of their hormone levels, creating "moobs" or man boobs, low mood, libido and sexual dysfunction.

Xenoestrogens are also present in:
- takeaway coffee cups and
- cling film (especially when heated)

Give me the drugs

During my nurse training, I learned that about 30% of the active ingredients in any drug we take, whether an over-the-counter or prescription medication or any supplement for that matter, is pee'd out of the body.

This means that we are all exposed to high levels of oestrogen in our drinking water that is being excreted by the many thousands of women who are taking HRT and the contraceptive pill. We are also being exposed to high levels of other drugs such as antidepressants (our birds and animals are exposed to these in the water supply too).

And of course any medication, even our most commonly prescribed or over the counter pharmaceutical drugs, act like toxins in the body and also affect the way our bodies can absorb essential nutrients from our foods.

The Heart of a Woman
How to look after the heart you give to the world - Gill Barham
pg. 46

It is a bit of a minefield isn't it?

What's going on inside?

So let's look now at the toxins that are coming from within – the **Endogenous toxins**.

Free radical damage comes from the process of oxidisation and is a big subject that is covered in chapter V. This is a natural ageing process but one that we would do well to control.

Faulty or bad gut bacteria can also be very toxic to the body and a recent study shows that simple things like saccharin and aspartame can interact with our gut bacteria and upset the balance.

However, the most exciting discovery to be made in recent years within the biomedical world, is the confirmation of the strength of the link between gut flora, known as the **microbiome** and the cause

The Heart of a Woman
How to look after the heart you give to the world - Gill Barham
pg. 47

and development of ill health, weight gain and disease. We look more closely at this in the next section.

"The microbiome has been dubbed "the forgotten organ," but I think it's high time doctors remembered it!"
Dr. Raphael Keliman

I am having fun …. But

A major cause of toxicity in our modern day lives is the high levels of the steroid hormones, adrenaline and cortisol that are produced as a result of stress.

Stress can be caused by pressure at work, emotional or relationships issues, what's happening at home, financial worries or even physical activity.

Stress can be perceived or unperceived.

I have been working with a lady recently who, when asked "do you have a stressful life" replied "no I really enjoy my job". However,
- she had a very high functioning role,
- she was under huge pressure to deliver a million-pound project,
- she exercised 3-4 times a week,

The Heart of a Woman
How to look after the heart you give to the world - Gill Barham
pg. 48

- she was driving 45 miles to and from work every day which could take anything from forty-five minutes to three hours,
- she was looking after an elderly relative at the weekends and
- she was struggling to eat a healthy diet.

PHEW!

So this "unperceived" stress was making her tired, overweight and prone to illness etc. Once we started working together, she realised that she needed a better work - lifestyle - nutrition balance and not only changed some lifestyle habits but lost 5kgs in 8 weeks in the process.

Outside v inside = same result
This build up, the combination of exogenous and endogenous toxins often results in diseases that are prevalent in the western world today.

Auto immune diseases:
- Fibromyalgia
- Chronic Fatigue Syndrome
- ME
- MS
- Rheumatoid arthritis
- Type 1 Diabetes

The Heart of a Woman
How to look after the heart you give to the world - Gill Barham
pg. 49

Endocrine disorders:

- Infertility
- PCOS
- PMS
- Menopausal symptoms
- Thyroid imbalances

Common disorders and complaints such as:

- Weight gain
- Insulin resistance/Diabetes (type 2)
- Headaches/migraines
- Joint pain
- IBS/digestive issues
- Cancer
- Heart disease
- Mental health problems
- Depression
- ADHD
- Learning disorders
- Parkinson's Disease
- Mood swings
- Panic attacks
- Memory loss

POPs and Diabetes – research study report in "Diabetes Care"

"….. these findings suggest that persistent organic pollutants - POPs may be associated with the risk of type 2 diabetes risk by increasing

The Heart of a Woman
How to look after the heart you give to the world - Gill Barham
pg. 50

insulin resistance and POPs may interact with obesity to further increase this risk"

Your fat is your friend.

THANK GOODNESS FOR FAT CELLS!

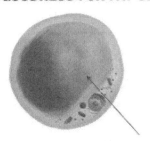

Toxins are stored within Fatty Tissue

When we are very chemically overloaded, when our bodies are very "toxic" we have this wonderful mechanism to keep our vital organs safe from these toxins. We store them in our fat cells. Now that means, that if your daily toxic overload is great, then you need more fat in order to store those toxins away.

Makes sense huh?

If each cell is covered in a bigger layer of fat, then the knock-on effect of this is that there are hormone disruptions and nutritional deficiencies. This is because
1. it's impossible for good things i.e. nutrition, to get through the cell wall but also
2. it's tricky to get the bad things, i.e. toxins, out.

The Heart of a Woman
How to look after the heart you give to the world - Gill Barham
pg. 51

This is one of the reasons it is so difficult for many people to lose weight, as the body will hold on to the fat for as long as these toxins need to be kept safely out of the way.

Here is a word that has been coined recently in the functional nutrition world to explain what is happening. This word is *obesogens*. These are chemicals that really shouldn't be there, that we should not be exposed to, that directly affect our fat stores by causing by this endocrine disruption.

Examples of Obesogens are:
- the POPs
- BPA's
- MSG
- Synthetic hormones - Xenoestrogens
- flame retardants – these have to be added to our clothes and to our soft furnishing by law.

In fact, I have a little story about this. My husband and I bought a mattress before one Christmas without realising that it was going to come chemically loaded with a flame retardant. It stank!! We had it in our bedroom for four weeks with the windows wide open before we could sleep on it.

The Heart of a Woman
How to look after the heart you give to the world - Gill Barham
pg. 52

So what is your "Chemical Cocktail"?

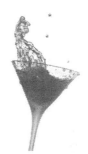

Can you see that it is not ONE toxin alone that is causing the diseases of today but the combination of toxins that are burdening the body?

So what is it that your body is being exposed to every day?

Is there a way in which you can minimise the exposure to this chemical overload and to the toxins that you are experiencing in our modern day world?

Perhaps you could grab a pen and paper and makes a note of the daily toxins that your body is exposed to?

The Heart of a Woman
How to look after the heart you give to the world - Gill Barham
pg. 53

"We have internal mechanisms designed to break down toxins but when the cocktail of chemicals over-whelm the body's detoxification mechanisms the body is in a critical situation"
Steven Horne

The Heart of a Woman
How to look after the heart you give to the world - Gill Barham
pg. 54

Is your body in a critical situation?

Have you come to the realisation, just like I did in 2012, that there are things that you've been exposed to that are affecting your health and even perhaps your weight?

What can we do about it? Well we can't hide away from the world, but we can minimise some of them, reduce the burden of the toxic load and help your system survive and thrive.

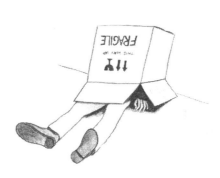

The Heart of a Woman
How to look after the heart you give to the world - Gill Barham
pg. 55

IV.2 CLEANSE & HEAL

Now that the importance of getting rid of the toxic load on our bodies is evident, once you get to grips with what you need to do to cleanse your body of these toxins you will always have a tool to fall back on that will help you to **purify**, **fortify** and **protect** your system at any time. You will always have the ability to know how you can help your body to detoxify and get rid of the chemical overload that we have identified and to restore balance and harmony particularly in your **microbiome.**

But without this, your body is always going to be suffering with that chemical overload. It is always going to be on the back foot, struggling to keep up with our 21st century living and it's more likely to succumb to disease, to weight gain, to premature aging and chronic illness and early death.

The science bit

ELITE HEALTH AND THE MICROBIOME

I am dedicated to helping you unlock your potential and achieve Elite Health. Elite Health is the pinnacle of wellness; where age does not dictate ability. It's about having the energy to push yourself to

- See more......
- Do more......and
- Be more.....no matter the stage of life you're in.

It's about stepping into every new decade with new ambition.

The Heart of a Woman
How to look after the heart you give to the world - Gill Barham
pg. 56

"Elite Health gives you the freedom to live without limitation, and it's through a healthy mind and body that this freedom is realised." Dr. Matt Tripp

The Heart of a Woman
How to look after the heart you give to the world - Gill Barham
pg. 57

How you achieve Elite Health begins with a focus on what makes every person unique and functional. You see, within each one of us, there is something particularly incredible going on that you may not realise. Your body is happily hosting 100 Trillion microorganisms. In other words, your body is a like a bustling city, home to a thriving community of microscopic, living, hard-working microbes.

In fact, only 10% of your body contains your DNA! The other 90% of you is bacteria, fungi, microflora, etc. That is YOUR microbiome. It's your "inner ecosystem" ...featuring over 10,000 identified species.

As these species are being further identified by science, and as the human microbiome is beginning to be explored, amazing things are being discovered and the buzz is building! It is truly an exciting time. And why is it exciting? Why are experts around the world so intensely focused on the microbiome? And why should we start to now care and think about the trillions of organisms living inside of us?

Because studies are showing that when you feed your microbiome the right way, and take care of your microbiome health, your body benefits in the most amazing, even surprising ways.

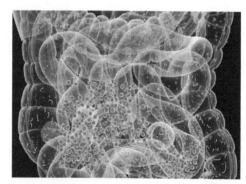

And it all starts inside your gut.

After all, it's the path taken by everything you've ever eaten or drunk. Your gut isn't just about digesting foods. It's home to billions of microbes, and these microbes can work for you, or against you. A healthy gut, made possible by a well-balanced microbiome, can lead to a variety of overall health benefits, including...
improved

- weight management,
- emotions,
- memory and
- immunity.

The gut microbiome is even connected to the health of neighbour organs, including your heart, skin, and reproductive system.

By eating to purify, fortify and protect your gut health, you'll be enhancing the overall social network of microbes alive inside you now. For too long the important bacteria within people has been ignored. Instead, temporary solutions and "bandage treatments" have become the norm, treatments that deal with what we now know to be merely symptoms of an imbalanced, impure microbiome.

With a focus on and understanding of, the root of our health, can we really transform the way we feel and function?

Experts are saying **yes**.

The Heart of a Woman
How to look after the heart you give to the world - Gill Barham
pg. 59

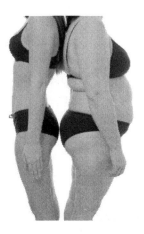

OBESE TWIN
BACTERIA
+ MOUSE
= **OBESE** MOUSE

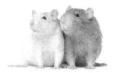

Consider a recent study conducted using four sets of twin sisters. In each set, one twin happened to be lean while the other was obese. Scientists carefully took intestinal bacteria from each sister, a sample of their microbiome, and implanted it into germ free mice... siblings of the same litter. The microbes from the gut of the lean sister were put into one mouse, and the mouse remained lean. On the other hand, the microbes that came from the gut of the obese sister dramatically affected their new host... the mouse got fat! Though both groups of mice exercised and were fed the same foods, the microbiome held the power to transform its host.

And it's a power over much more than just weight... it's about optimal metabolic function. It's about...ELITE HEALTH.

This study is just one of many. Experts throughout the world are now studying and experimenting with the microbiome, looking to

The Heart of a Woman
How to look after the heart you give to the world - Gill Barham
pg. 60

harness its power. One of those experts is Dr. Matthew Tripp, a pioneer in metabolic research. This Chief Scientific Officer continues a meritorious career of clinical trial, research, discovery and patents at the Hughes Center for Research and Innovation, where he and his team investigate the microbiome, test efficacious formulas, and oversee the scientific discovery and development of effective natural formulas that I use myself and recommend to others.

With the "first to market" highly sophisticated, clinically trialed "purify, fortify and protect" programmes that I am introducing my clients to, we really are ahead of the game in terms of achieving ELITE HEALTH.

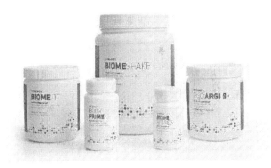

When I work with my clients, the first thing we address is re setting the microbiome incorporating my PURE 21 programme into the Healthy Starter Programme™ module.

This Lifestyle plan is patented and clinically trialled.

The Heart of a Woman
How to look after the heart you give to the world - Gill Barham
pg. 61

"So, we have just completed the 7-day microbiome reset week of the 21 day PURE 21 programme. I have been eating 3 healthy sugar free, wheat free meals a day with 1 shake mid-afternoon. My husband has followed the same plan but refused to give up his one coffee a day! I have added an extra 5,000 steps a day as the plan suggests. We have both lost just under 4 lbs which we hadn't shifted since our summer hols. I've had loads of energy, but Hubby has been a bit grumpy without his sugar fixes! Only negative side effect was a mild headache on the first day. The other positive is the eczema on my hand has almost disappeared"

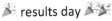 results day

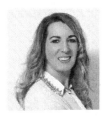
Completed my 7 days
Weight loss - 4lb 6oz
Waist - 1-inch loss
tummy - 1-inch loss
hips - 1-inch loss
bust - 1-inch loss 😫😪😵😵
Energy - through the roof all day long

Attitude - more positive and focused. Clear mind, also feel calmer

Sleep - very deep, no waking up for a wee as usual and waking up before my alarm clock (normally hate mornings)

Appetite - no hunger and no cravings. After day 3 I wasn't even missing my coffee. Had a chocolate cake on the kitchen side and normally I'd demolish it but wasn't tempted.

Side effects - mild niggly headache day 1-2 due to caffeine withdrawal I think. Stomach felt slight pain evening of day 1.

The Heart of a Woman
How to look after the heart you give to the world - Gill Barham
pg. 62

IV. 3 CARDIAC HEALTH

So, we have ARRIVED at the **HEART OF THE MATTER.**

When I trained as a nurse many years ago, I was expected to have an understanding of the disease process; rakes of terminology, technical terms associated with diagnostic procedures, surgery, medicine, drugs, and much more.

One of these terms was HOMEOSTASIS.

For the past 7 years, since I have been looking at health from a wellness perspective, rather than dealing with "DIS-EASE" or "illness", Homeostasis has become an ever-increasing focus of my work on my own health, and with that of my family, friends and many hundreds of clients.

Let's take a look at the 5 fundamentals that make up Homeostasis in the body.

1. Oxygen
2. Nutrients
3. Water
4. Regulated heat
5. Removal of waste

Each cell is reliant on a balance of all 5 elements and it is the imbalance or altered "Homeostasis" that is at the root of illness, ageing and ultimately death. So what system of the body is mostly responsible for homeostasis? What's the common denominator?

The Heart of a Woman
How to look after the heart you give to the world - Gill Barham
pg. 63

It's the Cardiovascular System.

It's a bit like a car. The engine has to be in good condition for efficiency, smooth running, and longevity of the vehicle. (This is why we spend money on servicing our cars to avoid breaking down and to get as much mileage as we can.)

Now, it is MY belief that we need to invest in a similar way to the maintenance of the engine of our "Cardiovascular System": your HEART, which beats an estimated 3.5 Million Times in a life-time, and your CIRCULATION.

We have already established that HEART DISEASE kills more men and women in the western world than Cancer, Diabetes, Respiratory Disease and Accidents combined.

Well this may be because the body's engine (heart) and cardiovascular (exhaust) system is clogged, out of condition, or over stressed.

Ageing, poor diet, lack of exercise, and conversely; inadequate nutrients to support exercise recovery, plus stress, disease, obesity may all lead to the four major risk factors of HEART DISEASE or STROKE.

1. **high blood pressure,**

2. **high cholesterol,**

3. **arteriosclerosis,**

4. **inflammation**:

The Heart of a Woman
How to look after the heart you give to the world - Gill Barham
pg. 64

Does it make sense to you then, that if you keep your body's engine and your exhaust system clean and strong that you will be less likely to experience a "car crash", a "break down" in other words a "FATALITY"?

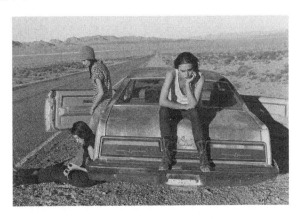

It does to me too.

So, what is the simplest, most effective, natural way to you ensure you keep your body strong and running smoothly? In the same way, as you would look after a car, by putting in good fuel and oil, you can help to make the next thousands of miles or ensure your life-times 3.5 million heartbeats.

Now, here's the exciting thing. If you get this right, you can not only prevent cardiovascular disease, but as you will see, you can also reverse it. You may be thinking; How is that possible?

It's time to introduce you to a "Miracle Molecule", NITRIC OXIDE (NO).

The Heart of a Woman
How to look after the heart you give to the world - Gill Barham
pg. 65

Nitric Oxide is the Body's "Miracle Molecule"

The discovery of this Miracle Molecule, is hailed as equally important to our nation's health as the discovery of X-rays, Insulin, Penicillin, Blood Groups, In Vitro Fertilisation, and Gene Therapy, the list goes on.

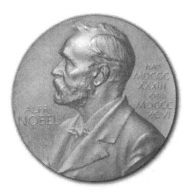

The Nobel Prize in Physiology or Medicine 1998

Awarded to: Robert F. Furchgott, Louis J. Ignarro and Ferid Murad

"for their discoveries concerning nitric oxide as a signaling molecule in the cardiovascular system"

The benefits of nitric oxide are many and they focus mainly in the cardio vascular system but this also impacts on other systems as well because nitric oxide can keep your blood vessels healthy by increasing blood flow. What happens is that the nitric oxide makes sure that all the organs in the body receive the normal amount of blood and therefore nutrients and oxygen that is required. In addition, nitric oxide can interfere with the blood clotting process

The Heart of a Woman
How to look after the heart you give to the world - Gill Barham
pg. 66

and so it can prevent unwanted blood clotting. When people suffer from a heart attack, in many cases this is due to a blood clot that develops in the coronary arteries that feed blood to the heart by the same mechanism. When a person gets a stroke, this is generally due to the development of a blood clot in the cerebral arteries that carry blood to the brain. The only time you want a blood clot to occur is when you injure yourself; you get a cut and you want a clot to form because that clot forms a plug and prevents the excessive loss of blood. However, you don't want those blood clots to occur in a normal artery in the brain or heart. So, nitric oxide is something we make to prevent that unwanted clotting of blood.

Memory and Learning

Our nerves stimulate different parts of the body. They do so by releasing a chemical. The major chemical in the brain that is released from many nerves is, guess what? Nitric oxide and this nitric oxide is well known today to facilitate memory and learning. Scientists have discovered that in memory and learning disorders, particularly **Alzheimer's disease**, there is a deficiency, often a marked deficiency in the formation of nitric oxide in those regions of the brain that regulate memory and learning. Infact several pharmaceutical companies have developed drugs that stimulate nitric oxide formation in those regions of the brain and the early clinical studies show that if you boost nitric oxide formation in the brain you can restore memory and learning. So, there is hope for everyone who is suffering from a memory and learning disorder.

The Heart of a Woman
How to look after the heart you give to the world - Gill Barham
pg. 67

Normal service is resumed

Not only does this nitric oxide decrease the blood pressure and protect against heart disease one of the major effects of nitric oxide in the body is to function as a vasodilator. This means it is going to widen or relax the arteries and when that happens you are going to increase the flow of blood to the "other end". Dr Ignarro and his colleagues made an interesting discovery back in 1990 when they showed that the nerves that go to the erectile tissue of men **and women** actually release nitric oxide as the signalling molecule or neurotransmitter.

Before they made that discovery, the neurotransmitter was not known and if you don't know what the nerves are releasing to stimulate a function it's almost impossible to develop a rational drug to treat a disease. Do you see? As a result, for many years most sexual dysfunction and lack of libido was put down to psychological issues. Once scientists showed that those nerves release nitric oxide, one of the pharmaceutical companies developed a big programme to look at that. They extended Dr Ignarro's research further and *voilà!* they came up with the drug Viagra which is the first orally available drug that is useful in treating impotence or erectile dysfunction. The way Viagra works is simply to enhance and increase the actions of nitric oxide. For any couple that have issues in this area, and this is much more common than you may expect, the ability to be able to understand how to **improve libido** and sexual function is critical for a happy, healthy sex-life, and therefore a fulfilling and long lasting relationship.

The Heart of a Woman
How to look after the heart you give to the world - Gill Barham
pg. 68

Dr. Louis Ignarro is a distinguished Professor of Pharmacology at the UCLA School of Medicine and has spent 30 years of his life researching how to improve heart health without prescription drugs and is the author of the book NO More Heart Disease...How Nitric Oxide Can Prevent Even Reverse Heart Disease and Strokes.

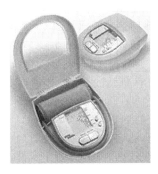

No pressure!

Nitric oxide is a vasodilator which means it's going to widen blood vessels and lower the pressure within the blood vessels. What is interesting is that it doesn't lower blood pressure if the blood pressure is normal. This is the beauty about the natural substances present in our body. Nitric oxide senses when the blood pressure is abnormally elevated and then it steps in to reduce that blood pressure back down to the normal range, **but not below normal**. It is the most effective substance we have in the body, the most effective hormone to lower the blood pressure and keep it out of the high range. It is something that you want to do all the time, you want to have sufficient amounts of nitric oxide around consistently to keep that blood pressure down, because high blood pressure can lead to a heart attack or stroke.

The Heart of a Woman
How to look after the heart you give to the world - Gill Barham

"The single most common cause of cardiovascular disease is a persistent high blood pressure that the person does not control".
Dr Ignarro

The Heart of a Woman
How to look after the heart you give to the world - Gill Barham
pg. 70

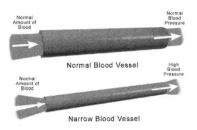

Normal Amount of Blood

Normal Blood Pressure

Normal Blood Vessel

High Blood Pressure

Normal Amount of Blood

Narrow Blood Vessel

Blood Pressure Blood Flow

This is because that pressure against the arteries will eventually tear apart the cells, rip apart the arterial cells and this is going to cause irreversible damage to the arteries, especially the development of plaque formation and cholesterol build-up in the arteries. This will begin to precipitate blood clotting which means you can get a blood clot on the heart precipitating a heart attack, a blood clot in the brain which will cause a stroke or a blood clot to the lung which is also fatal, and was the cause of my Mother's premature death.

So, nitric oxide is the body's natural way to prevent all of these things from happening. One of the most common causes of a heart attack or stroke is the development of atherosclerosis , simply an inflammatory disease of the arteries and this comes about when you have cholesterol build-up, in other words a bad cholesterol or LDL cholesterol build-up. This will actually cause a change in the structure of the arteries; the blood will begin to clot, there will be all kinds of debris clinging to one another and this constitutes the build-up of plaque in the arterial wall which can obstruct blood flow.

The Heart of a Woman
How to look after the heart you give to the world - Gill Barham
pg. 71

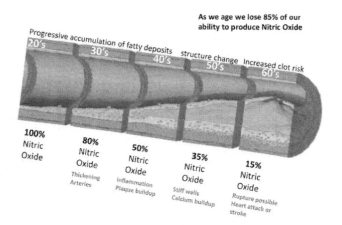

As we age we lose 85% of our ability to produce Nitric Oxide

Progressive accumulation of fatty deposits

structure change   Increased clot risk

20's   30's   40's   50's   60's

100% Nitric Oxide

80% Nitric Oxide

Thickening Arteries

50% Nitric Oxide

Inflammation Plaque buildup

35% Nitric Oxide

Stiff walls Calcium buildup

15% Nitric Oxide

Rupture possible Heart attack or stroke

Worse yet if those plaques become disrupted for any reason, they too can travel to different parts of the body causing heart attacks or strokes. The way the body protects naturally against the development of high cholesterol is through NO = nitric oxide. Nitric oxide functions to keep the balance of the various lipids in in the arterial system so it helps to maintain the good cholesterol and the bad cholesterol at healthy levels.

Some of our very famous drugs, the statin drugs that are made by many different companies are great at reducing your bad cholesterol. The way those statins work is by stimulating nitric oxide formation in the arteries, so if you have sufficient amounts of nitric oxide in your healthy arteries you don't have to take statin drugs.

The Heart of a Woman
How to look after the heart you give to the world - Gill Barham
pg. 72

I have included a bonus for you of an episode of "Gill Barham - The Miracle Molecule Host" in conversation with Marina Nani – of Radio W.O.R.K.S. World. Listen in to the **Facts and Myths about cholesterol and statins episode.**

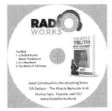 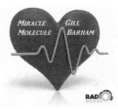

Mr Nobel's heart.

The most common medication given to relieve the symptoms of chest pain or angina is GTN, nitro-glycerine. How ironic that 100 years earlier, when Alfred Nobel, the creator of both dynamite and the Nobel Prize, was taken ill with heart disease...his doctor prescribed for him nitro-glycerine, which he refused to take. But 100 years later, the nitro-glycerine in his dynamite actually led to his Nobel Prize being awarded for the discovery that nitric oxide is the gas molecule released in the nitro-glycerine that has the life-saving effect of increasing blood flow and preventing a heart attack. It is documented that his factory workers reported that their angina pain would subside on weekdays when they were exposed to nitro-glycerine fumes, only to worsen at the weekends.

Say YES to NO.

The Heart of a Woman
How to look after the heart you give to the world - Gill Barham

My clients have access to the most effective and most natural way possible to increase NO (nitric oxide) in the body on a consistent level. Through a combination of NO enhancing foods and the only patent pending dietary supplement available today, **Proargi9+** we are seeing the most amazing results.

Case study

*Angela is 64, slim and outwardly healthy and she has very regular health checks as she is part of the Great Ormond Street Twins Study. She was aware of a tendency to a slightly **high blood pressure**, particularly if taken by a medical professional, (white coat syndrome) and was due to see her GP in about 2 weeks or so who she thought would want her to take medication. We did Angela's Tamah (Arterial Stiffness) test as part of a routine health check and we were both very concerned by the results. Angela had **no symptom**s of a struggling cardiovascular system, is of a normal weight, eats a very healthy diet and takes fairly regular exercise. She does, however have a long history of **familial heart attacks** on her father's side.*

*As Angela wanted to avoid taking the BP medication and Statins that her GP wanted to prescribe for her, I recommended that Angela try upping her production of NO, The Miracle Molecule, with the patented product called **ProArgi9+**.*

The Heart of a Woman
How to look after the heart you give to the world - Gill Barham
pg. 74

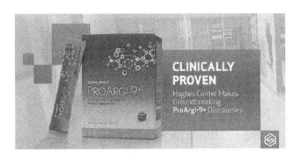

The following images are the representations of Angela's progress over just 3 months of taking **ProArgi9**+ The results are the average of 3 readings of the LAST TEST. (Her BP at the first readings were over the threshold for the chart and were actually much higher 200/97). She did not change her diet or her lifestyle over the 3 months between tests.

Biological age dropped from 79 - 61

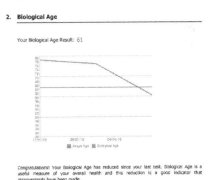

2. **Biological Age**

Your Biological Age Result: 61

Congratulations! Your Biological Age has reduced since your last test. Biological Age is a useful measure of your overall health and this reduction is a good indicator that improvements have been made.

The Heart of a Woman
How to look after the heart you give to the world - Gill Barham

Blood pressure dropped from 200/97 to 148/87 (the initial readings were off the chart)

---

5. Blood Pressure

Your Blood Pressure reading for this test: 148/87

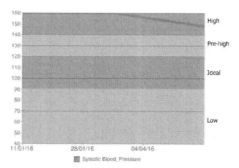

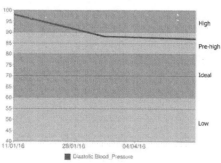

Your reading indicates that you may have high blood pressure (hypertension). You should consult with your doctor or nurse. Also you may be able to make some lifestyle changes to help lower your blood pressure.

The Heart of a Woman
How to look after the heart you give to the world - Gill Barham

Arterial Stiffness dropped from 8 (highest level) to 2

3. Arterial Stiffness

Your Arterial Stiffness Index reading for this test: 2

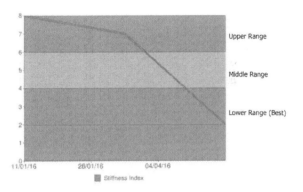

The TAMAH procedure is a test of the endothelial function and elasticity of your arteries and expresses this as arterial stiffness. If the endothelium does not work properly, this can be associated with a condition called endothelium dysfunction which results in a loss of elasticity or the artery described above. This dysfunction has now been seen as a precursor to the development of ischaemic heart disease (narrowing of the heart arteries with fat) and strokes.

Your arterial stiffness has reduced since your last visit. This is an excellent result and demonstrates how valuable it is to pay continued attention to your health in terms of arterial stiffness. You may be able to improve this result still further by continuing to eat a healthy diet, getting plenty of exercise and making sure you have adequate hydration.

We would ask you to remember that all of the results within this report are to be used as a guide and for reference only. The results are not intended as a diagnosis.

Angela is continuing with her ProArgi9+ sachets and is feeling much happier and more confident about her future with her new husband.

The Heart of a Woman
How to look after the heart you give to the world - Gill Barham
pg. 77

Here is a list of the NO producing foods that I recommended for Angela to boost NO production alongside her therapeutic supplement regime.

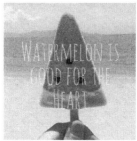

Water melon is great as it the source of L-Citrulline, the amino acid that helps with the production of NO in the body.

Garlic: Lowers blood pressure and cholesterol, as well as reducing the stickiness of the blood. Eat at least one whole clove daily in food.

Parsley: Protects against high blood pressure through its diuretic activities.

All the berries: Anti-oxidant and heart-protective, so use regularly (I a drink which has the antioxidant equivalent of 3.5kg of fruit in one 30ml shot!!)

Apples: Two a day can help lower cholesterol levels

Beans: Provide soluble fibre which lowers cholesterol.

Oatmeal: Contains soluble fibre and Vitamin E for a healthy heart.

Whitebait: Like all oily fish, contains heart protective fatty acids but no damaging saturated fats.

So why should I care about my arterial age?

The Heart of a Woman
How to look after the heart you give to the world - Gill Barham
pg. 78

The age of your arteries is directly or indirectly implicated in practically **every cellular response** and health condition imaginable

- **cardiovascular** system
- **immune** system,
- **hormone** function
- **nerve** and **brain** function
- **skin and joints**
- **gut** function
- **sexual** function
- **kidney** function

The following are the *22* primary **scientifically backed** reasons that anyone, **even healthy people**, should consider adding the amino acids L-arginine and L-citrulline to their health and wellness regime.

RESEARCH HAS SHOWN THAT L-ARGININE

1 – is **one thousand times** more powerful than any naturally occurring **antioxidant** in the body and may protect against **heart disease**, **stroke, cancer,** and **diabetes**, as well as slowing premature **ageing.**

2 – offers wide-ranging cardiovascular support, including **controlling blood pressure** and **plaque** formation helps normalise blood pressure, preventing hypertension and **angina.**

3 – enhances **memory**, may help to reverse the effects of **dementia** and **Alzheimer's** disease.

The Heart of a Woman
How to look after the heart you give to the world - Gill Barham
pg. 79

4 – boosts human growth hormone (**HGH**) production, which has **anti-aging** properties.

5 – enhances messages between **nerves** and the **brain.**

6 – may help improve **immune** function and fight **bacterial infections.**

7 – may help in the treatment and complications of **diabetes** including **poor circulation and blindness,** and is also found to **regulate insulin** secretion in the pancreas.

8 – may inhibit the division and proliferation of **cancer** cells.

9 – helps with **cholesterol** control by lowering serum and LDL cholesterol levels.

10 – enhances male sexual performance by treating vascular **erectile dysfunction** (ED).

11 – anticoagulant abilities reduce clotting to **lower heart attack** and **stroke risk.**

12 – reduces **pregnancy-related hypertension**, a risk factor for both the expecting mother and the unborn child.

13 – is useful in the treatment of **asthma** and the treatment of lung disorders.

14 – relaxes hypertonic sphincter muscles, preventing and healing **hemorrhoids.**

15 – boosts lean muscle mass and preserves bone density so it may be useful in **weight management** and **strength training.**

16 – boosts nitric oxide levels in **smokers**

17 – helps to accelerate **wound healing, post-surgery recovery, burns especially** in the **elderly.**

18 – enhances **athletic performance** due to its ability to boost exercise tolerance, and build lean muscle tissue.

19 – may be used to improve the function of the **prostate.**

20 – may prevent and possible reverse the effects of **osteoporosis**

21 – has been used in the treatment of **irritable bowel syndrome** and to reduce the occurrence of **ulcers** (especially stress-related) without affecting gastric acid production.

22 – may improve **kidney function** and slow the progression of renal disease and age-related chronic renal failure. L-arginine's protective effect on the kidneys may also benefit those with diabetes.

The more we can work towards a healthy lifestyle the better chance we have of avoiding a catastrophe. Eating well, taking moderate exercise, reducing stress, creating a good work/life balance will increase your sense of well-being, but **ProArgi9+** is the fuel, oil, air, water and pump primer that will make you feel like a high performance car rather than the slightly neglected vehicle that may just be on the brink of a breakdown.

So you can see how we can help to save 1 Million Lives a Year with the Miracle Molecule.

The Heart of a Woman
How to look after the heart you give to the world - Gill Barham
pg. 81

"I have saved the lives of 150 people from heart transplantations. If I had focused on preventive medicine earlier, I would have saved 150 million."

Christiaan Barnard

CHAPTER V

Prevent

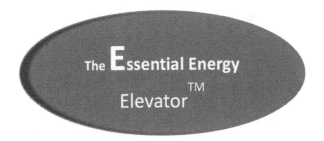

V. 1 FLUID

This is the life blood of your body. Your body can only function if it is hydrated and as adults we are made up of 60-75% water.

It is recommended that we drink an average of 2 litres of filtered water a day; (you know already why it needs to be filtered right?) less or more depending on whether you are a small or larger lady.

That does not include the water in your beverages or squashes etc. (Although I do count it in my fruit or herbal teas).

The Heart of a Woman
How to look after the heart you give to the world - Gill Barham
pg. 83

Here are the top 10 functions of water in your body

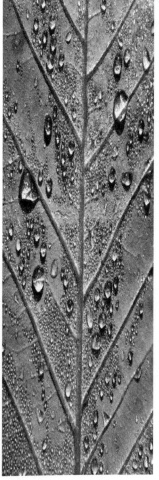

Moistens tissues such as those in the mouth eyes and nose

Protects body organs and tissues

Helps prevent constipation

Helps dissolve minerals and other nutrients to make the accessible to the body

Regulates body temperature

Lubricates joints

Lessens the burden on the kidneys and liver by flushing out waste products

Carries nutrients and oxygen to the cells

Aids in weight loss

Ensures a healthy cardiovascular system

The Heart of a Woman
How to look after the heart you give to the world - Gill Barham
pg. 84

If you are dehydrated then you will notice it has an influence on all of your systems, including your cardiovascular system, your brain function, your gut function, your skeletal system; i.e. your skin, your joints and your spine.

Here are some common signs that you may not be drinking enough:

- Headaches
- Painful joints
- Backache
- Depression
- High blood pressure
- Allergies
- Digestive problems
- Difficulties in concentration
- Symptoms of memory loss

Let's look at an example.

There are discs that sit in between all the bones in your spine and they are there to support the vertebra. These intervertebral discs are also made up of 60-75% water, so if you are dehydrated then your spine will be less mobile and less healthy.

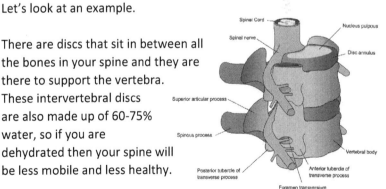

The Heart of a Woman
How to look after the heart you give to the world - Gill Barham
pg. 85

As a Pilates teacher, what I see regularly is that not drinking enough water is one of the most common reasons for back pain.

Here's the thing...

If you are thirsty, you are already dehydrated!

www.theLifestyleLeader.co.uk

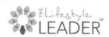

The Heart of a Woman
How to look after the heart you give to the world - Gill Barham
pg. 86

What else should I drink and what should I avoid?

There is much evidence that eating and drinking green juices that alkalise the body are beneficial to good health. Starting the day with a slice of lemon in warm water is a great start, as is adding a liquid chlorophyll concentrate to your water throughout the day. (I am slightly addicted to this stuff to be honest!) Be careful with lemon water though, as too much can damage your teeth.

It is important to have an alkaline pH in your body, because it has been found that in an over-acid state, bacteria, viruses, fungi, and even cancer cells can grow faster.

90% of people have over acidic bodies, because we don't get enough natural green nutrition in our modern diets and we eat too many acid forming foods:

pH	Acidic	pH SPECTRUM	Alkaline	pH

			Neutral pH	
3	Carbonated Water, Club Soda, Energy Drinks	7	Most Tap Water, Most Spring Water, Sea Water, River Water	
4	Popcorn, Cream Cheese, Buttermilk, Prunes, Pastries, Pasta, Cheese, Pork, Beer, Wine, Black Tea, Pickles, Chocolate, Roasted Nuts, Vinegar, Sweet and Low, Equal, Nutra Sweet	8	Apples, Almonds, Tomatoes, Grapefruit, Corn, Mushrooms, Turnip, Olive, Soybeans, Peaches, Bell Pepper, Radish, Pineapple, Cherries, Wild Rice, Apricot, Strawberries, Bananas	
5	Most Purified Water, Distilled Water, Coffee, Sweetened Fruit Juice, Pistachios, Beef, White Bread, Peanuts, Nuts, Wheat	9	Avocados, Green Tea, Lettuce, Celery, Peas, Sweet Potatoes, Egg Plant, Green Beans, Beets, Blueberries, Pears, Grapes, Kiwi, Melons, Tangerines, Figs, Dates, Mangoes, Papayas	
6	Fruit Juices, Most Grains, Eggs, Fish, Tea, Cooked Beans, Cooked Spinach, Soy Milk, Coconut, Lima Beans, Plums, Brown Rice, Barley, Cocoa, Oats, Liver, Oyster, Salmon	10	Spinach, Broccoli, Artichoke, Brussel Sprouts, Cabbage, Cauliflower, Carrots, Cucumbers, Lemons, Limes, Seaweed, Asparagus, Kale, Radish, Collard Greens, Onion	

The Heart of a Woman
How to look after the heart you give to the world - Gill Barham

Chlorophyll is a powerful alkaliser that helps raise your body's pH. A Nobel Prize in Chemistry was awarded to the German chemist, Richard Willstatter, for his studies on Chlorophyll.

Benefits of Liquid Chlorophyll:
Helps the body to stay alkaline
Blood cleansing
Immune enhancement
Increased intestinal health
Cardiovascular support
Chlorophyll is a great addition to maintain a healthy lifestyle, along with exercise and a balanced diet, I use one that is a rich source of alkaline substances from plant extracts such as barley grass, alfalfa and peppermint which I add to water.

So what's the big deal about caffeine?

Caffeine is a natural substance found in coffee beans, green tea, yerba matte, kola nuts, guarana seeds, and cola. Most people drink caffeine to wake them up, or keep them awake as it is a stimulant and this is a remedy for fatigue.

However, what is happening is all to do with the receptors in your brain. As you become tired, these receptors normally tell you that you need to rest, but caffeine blocks this effect by increasing levels of adrenaline and cortisol to keep you going. Now, you already know that these two stress hormones act as toxins in the body. But caffeine does not give you energy, it merely blocks the messages that you need to rest. There are times, clearly when that can be

The Heart of a Woman
How to look after the heart you give to the world - Gill Barham
pg. 88

handy!! However, when you use caffeine every day, the body produces more of these receptors in the hope that you may rest. So then you need the caffeine to maintain normal energy levels and you need to increase the dose in order to get the effect you want.

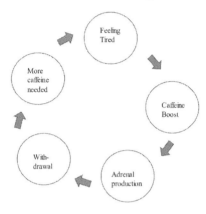

If you stop using caffeine, you will experience healing symptoms and withdrawal. However, the body will adjust these receptors downwards so that you can ultimately achieve a better balance.

To be honest, most drugs work in the body in the same way, which is why they are good for short term relief but not for long term use.

Ok so can I have a drink?

Yes, and it's like everything in life, moderation is key. You will be aware of the high amounts of sugar in alcohol and therefore the effect it will have on your weight, your acid/alkaline balance, your

The Heart of a Woman
How to look after the heart you give to the world - Gill Barham
pg: 89

kidney and liver function oh... and of course what it does to your brain!!

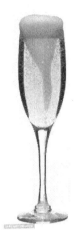

But a little of what you fancy does you good and I am not here to preach... indeed I love a Campari and Soda and would probably race you to the bar for a glass of champagne anytime!

The Heart of a Woman
How to look after the heart you give to the world - Gill Barham
pg. 90

V.2 FUNCTION

Let's take a look at how clever your body is! For most of the time, we take it for granted that our bodies will perform at the level we require to undertake whatever tasks we set for it. It adapts to temperatures, will keep us safe from harm and sometimes will even produce another little human being.

When it is in trouble though, it will tell you!

Our job is to listen …….. but most of us are rubbish at that!
Let's compare your body again to a car. Have you ever experienced seeing the lights flashing on the dashboard? These are warning lights that tell you if you need to do things like:
- Re-fuel
- Add more water to the windscreen or radiator
- Pump up the tyres
- Top up with oil
- Check the braking system
- Charge the air-con

I heard a radio programme recently where a gentleman told the presenter that he puts a sock in front of his dashboard so that he cannot see the warning lights!!

Would you agree with me that this would be totally foolish?
Well, I would suggest that this is exactly what we do all the time. The symptoms that show up for us are like the flashing lights on the car dashboard.

The Heart of a Woman
How to look after the heart you give to the world - Gill Barham
pg. 91

You could be experiencing such things as:

- Headaches
- Period pains
- Muscle cramps or joint aches
- Sleep disturbances
- Hormonal issues
- Weight gain or weight loss
- Lack of energy
- Digestive issues
- Low mood
- Depression or anxiety
- Memory loss or confusion
- High blood pressure
- Raised cholesterol levels
- Breathing difficulties

If, like me, you ignore the first warning light or lights, then your body will flash up another light, in other words another symptom and this will keep going until you either;

1. acknowledge the signs and take appropriate action or
2. develop a more serious condition or illness.

Do you remember we talked about taking care of the engine in your car? (e.g. your heart) Well, maybe not so much when I was younger, but now we also regularly commit to spending time and money on our family car; on the upholstery, paintwork, tyres, getting it cleaned and polished, fulfilling the basic needs in terms of fuel, oil and water the brakes, balancing the wheels and getting it regularly serviced.

The Heart of a Woman
How to look after the heart you give to the world - Gill Barham
pg. 92

My question to you is: Are you looking after your body in a similar fashion? Are you noticing when you experience symptoms and signs of illness or disease? What is your normal reaction to this?

You may be exactly like me when I had ignored the variety of symptoms for the two years that led to that lightbulb moment in November 2012. You may also look back "in hindsight" and notice what you have been experiencing lately or even over a longer period that has led to the point at which you are now.

My clients have the opportunity to really look at their present state of health with my help on The **Your H.E.A.R.T. Matters™** programme with a wellbeing questionnaire. I have included this in a later chapter for you to complete.

Let's talk about exercise.

There is no doubt that our sedentary lifestyles have an increasing impact on the state of the nation's health and the rise in the disease mega-trends of today.

I love the fact though that our modern-day world provides us with technology that gives us at least a helping hand and some motivation to get moving more. We can wear a clever bit of kit like a watch to monitor how much we move and even our smart phones can tell us what to eat, when to eat, how much sleep we are getting and how many flights of stairs we may have climbed in a day. There are so many health apps available to us and it is a great thing that

The Heart of a Woman
How to look after the heart you give to the world - Gill Barham
pg. 93

the government are funding projects that promote community sport and recreation activities to all.

All you need to do really, is find something that you love to do, or even a range of things to do, so that you don't get bored and if you can do it with friends, all the better.

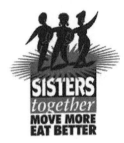

At the very least, try to walk 5,000 steps a day (that's twice around the field with the dogs for me) and if you can make 10,000, all the better.

We live in the middle of the countryside and have at least 50 – 100 cyclists pass the house most days .... yes even in winter ... and yes everyone is in lycra! That's not my bag and neither is running, but it may rock your boat. If so, that's great but .....

Ageing and exercise.

Whilst I do advocate exercise for all, it comes with a proviso. The more you exercise the more nutrition you need; especially in terms of antioxidants. If you exercise to get your heart rate up in any way, or you lift weights for example, you will be producing more free radicals in the body. Free radicals are what make us age inside and out and this is why we need to add extra nutrition in the form of antioxidants to our daily diet. This is covered in the next section.

The Heart of a Woman
How to look after the heart you give to the world - Gill Barham
pg. 94

"Those who think they have no time for bodily exercise will sooner or later have to find time for illness."

Edward Stanley

British statesman

The Heart of a Woman
How to look after the heart you give to the world - Gill Barham
pg. 95

V. 3 FIVE A DAY

Your body needs a range of nutrients every day.

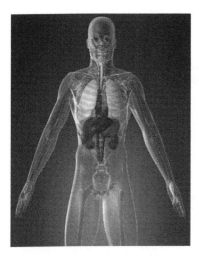

- Air
- Water
- Nutrition
  - Minerals
  - Vitamins
  - Antioxidants
  - Protein
  - Carbohydrates
  - Essential Fatty Acids
  - Enzymes
  - Phytonutrients
- Exercise
- Rest

Remind Me ... What Are Antioxidants and Why Do I Care?

We hear a lot about how antioxidants are great, but what does "antioxidant" even mean?

Well let's look first at the term "oxidant".

Oxidants are normal by-products of regular metabolism. As you break down food for energy and go about your life – even reading

The Heart of a Woman
How to look after the heart you give to the world - Gill Barham
pg. 96

this book - you are making oxidants. Bite into an apple and you will see oxidation in process as the flesh goes brown.

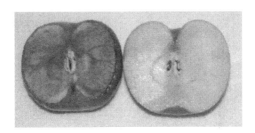

This same process is happening to us all on the outside, (visible by our wrinkles, lines, age spots etc.,) and of course... also on the inside! (If you paint the apple with lemon juice, the flesh stays healthy. This is because of the vitamin c in the lemon juice which is an antioxidant.)

Oxidants carry around an un-paired, or "free" electron and because of this electron, they have a negative charge and are sometimes also called "free radicals." Heard of them?

The body is happy when, on the whole, these negative charges pair off with positive ones and become neutral. In some cases, though, the free radicals don't get paired off, and these free electrons make a real nuisance of themselves by causing damage!

Now, in some cases the damage has a purpose.
i.e. one of the ways your immune system fights invaders and gets rid of damaged tissues is to produce free radicals that are powerfully destructive.

The Heart of a Woman
How to look after the heart you give to the world - Gill Barham

However, TOO MANY free radicals floating around, will damage the healthy parts of your body they come in contact with.

It is free radicals that switch on CANCER cells, and they also play a role in things like:
- heart disease,
- stroke,
- arthritis,
- alcoholic liver damage
- the ageing process.

Luckily, your body has a built-in defence system of antioxidants, molecules that scavenge and neutralise oxidants and often turn them into harmless oxygen and water.

However, your body will be overwhelmed and unable to manage excess free radicals under certain circumstances:

- chronic disease like diabetes, lupus, ME
- wear and tear on your body from a trauma (think a wound, break or an ACL tear)
- overuse (think tennis elbow),
- cigarette smoking
- alcohol
- consuming processed foods, fizzy drinks, (both examples of toxic stresses that rev up your immune system.)
- Stress

The Heart of a Woman
How to look after the heart you give to the world - Gill Barham
pg. 98

And when you undertake strenuous exercise!! How ironic is that?

There are certain stages in your life when some forms of exercise are more beneficial than others. This is covered in chapter VI.

So, this is why we care so much about antioxidants as they counteract the effects of free radical damage and will help us to keep well, free from colds, and flu, have more energy, clarity of thought, look younger and achieve optimum health.

You can find them in many foods, including:

almonds
spices (oregano, clove, turmeric, coriander, cilantro, cinnamon, ginger, dill, and others)
beans (red, kidney and pinto)
berries (cranberries, pomegranate seeds, blackberries and blueberries)
vegetables.

To get more antioxidants, easy ways are to:

1. Eat the rainbow; meaning consume a lot of brightly coloured fruits and vegetables.

2. Cook with spices.

3. Supplement with a high quality anti-oxidant as extra insurance, as we never, EVER catch up on the "bad" days!

The Heart of a Woman
How to look after the heart you give to the world - Gill Barham
pg. 99

Just one capful of the one I use contains the equivalent of 3.5 kilos of fruit. (If I ate the equivalent amount of fruit I would be consuming around 42 teaspoons of sugar!)

So, what else?

In the Your H.E.A.R.T. Matters™ programme my clients also learn about clean eating and how to balance the amounts of nutrients needed to maintain a healthy body. They learn how to ditch the processed foods in exchange for easy, tasty meals that are based on the highest quality fresh ingredients that are within their budget and freely available.

Achieving Elite Health is really all about being organised and changing habits... little by little.

By understanding some simple guidelines, it makes it easier to shop and plan for meals and will save money too!

If you just remember only to buy food with one ingredient you will not go far wrong. What do I mean? Have your lasagna but make it from fresh ingredients, that means ditching the bottled tomato pasta sauce that is full of additives and tons of sugar!

Did you know that MARS owns Dolmio sauces? Their latest marketing campaign addresses the upcoming sugar tax by advising that we only eat the product once a week. They are not reducing the sugar content though. More on that in the next chapter.

The Heart of a Woman
How to look after the heart you give to the world - Gill Barham
pg. 100

"Real food doesn't have ingredients; real food is ingredients"

Jamie Oliver

Chef and Author

CHAPTER VI

Perfect

The greatest gift I can give you is to help you to understand the difference between the most common type of health care in the western world; disease management and symptomatic relief, versus some more proactive and safer ways to achieve Elite Health. If like me, you live in the UK, then we benefit from our glorious NHS, but wherever you live you may choose, or be forced, to contribute to your own and your family's health financially. Whatever your access to health-care, I am guessing that it is based on the diagnosis of disease and the prescription of drug therapies. Western Medics and GP's are trained to do just that, but it wasn't always the case.

In the early twentieth century most medicines that people bought from the pharmacy were made by the pharmacist. The shelves around the shop were filled with ingredients to make all kinds of remedies. Customers could buy many medicines directly from the pharmacist. For others, a prescription was written by the doctor to tell the pharmacist what was required for the patient. Prescriptions were written in abbreviated medical Latin, so what the doctor prescribed was a mystery to the patient, a secret between him and the pharmacist. The only information given to the patient would be the dosage.

The Heart of a Woman
How to look after the heart you give to the world - Gill Barham
pg. 102

Our health care nowadays is driven by the big pharmaceutical companies. The medical profession as a whole is influenced in a big way, sadly, resulting in 2015 to 13 billion dollars in fines being issued to big US Pharma for bribing doctors to prescribe their drugs.

I want help my clients to avoid "the poly-pharmacy": the slippery slope of taking medicines without proper supervision or review. I saw a new Pilates client just recently who takes blood pressure pills, even though her BP is lower than normal, statins and dispersible aspirin every day. She has been doing this for years, without any review from her GP. When I asked her why she was still taking them, she didn't know.

So I believe that we should all be looking at an alternate NHS: Natural Health Solutions.

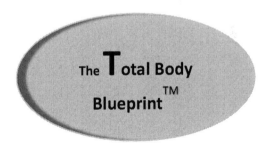

The Heart of a Woman
How to look after the heart you give to the world - Gill Barham
pg. 103

VI.1 Blood Sugar Balance

Sounds good but……. WHY do we need to do this?

As we have already established, the Low Fat diets introduced by Ancel Keys in the 1960's, whilst initially showing some success because it meant a change of habits back to healthier foods, with less saturated fats and sugar, actually became the downfall of calorie controlled dieting in the 1980's and onwards. This was because of the development and marketing of Low Fat Foods. These foods invariably have a higher sugar content to make up for the lower fat and therefore poorer taste. Foods that convert to sugar quickly have an acidic effect in the body and also an inflammatory effect. Neither of which are good for achieving or maintaining elite health. The recent acceptance of these effects on the body by the medical profession has led to new moves to reduce the epidemic of obesity and its effects on health by promoting healthier lifestyles, a more specifically a reduced consumption of processed foods and beverages that are high in sugar.

What's all the fuss?

The UK government announcement in 2016 that they will be introducing a sugar tax was a bit of a shocker, even for our very own celebrity campaigner Jamie Oliver. On the face of it, there is no doubt that sugar has a major effect on the nation's health, particularly in regard to the biggest killer, heart disease. Sugar's inflammatory properties are at the root of so many diseases and chronic illnesses of the 21st century, however I have been considering the pros and cons of this bold move!

The Heart of a Woman
How to look after the heart you give to the world - Gill Barham
pg. 104

Good... Taxing the manufacturers will force them to look at reducing the sugar content in drinks
Better. Education has to be the real key to long term change.
Bad...I do think this tax will affect the poor more than the wealthier UK citizens

Good ... Monies accrued will be used for sport in schools
Better. I would prefer to see this money spent on educating parents and children on healthy eating and cooking fresh food.
Bad. The cost of fresh food is also rising... Could we use the money to subsidise healthy, high quality food?

Good. Taxing sugar raises the profile of the effects that it food has on your health
Better... The majority of sugar consumption for the average person is through FOOD that had hidden sugars, so I think a tax on PROCESSED foods would be more effective.
Bad... My real concern is that there will be a switch to "diet" sodas, which are equally, if not MORE damaging to health due to the artificial sweeteners, such as Aspartame. (It's a bit like swapping heroin for methadone).

On balance, this is at the very least, the start of a campaign which we desperately need to reduce obesity, diabetes and heart disease rates in the UK. I do believe though that it is OUR responsibility to choose food that nourishes and builds health, not the job of government.

The Heart of a Woman
How to look after the heart you give to the world - Gill Barham
pg. 105

What is making us fat sick and tired?

Working with my clients over the years, one of the biggest problems in maintaining a healthy weight and therefore reducing the risk of obesity and the many associated health problems is understanding how to balance blood sugar levels in the body.

Is it just the white stuff?

When I talk about **sugar** I am referring to all foods that have high levels of added sugar as an ingredient or that convert to sugar very quickly. This is in addition to the sugar that you add to your food or beverages. These include:

- White breads, pasta, rice
- Cakes, biscuits
- Pastries – sweet and savoury
- Alcohol
- Squashes, cordials, sodas
- Bottled sauces, condiments
- Most breakfast cereals
- Sweets and ice creams
- Low fat foods

Very often it is the hidden sugars in foods that are a surprise to my clients who are trying to stop cravings, have more energy or avoid weight gain.

The problem with a diet that is high in sugary foods is the risk of "insulin resistance", "pre-diabetic state" and "Type II diabetes" which, guess what, all increase your risk of CADIOVASCULAR DISEASE.

The Heart of a Woman
How to look after the heart you give to the world - Gill Barham

Diabetes.

As part of the **Your H.E.A.R.T. Matters™** Programme, we take a journey into what the different types of diabetes are, how to prevent and reverse type II diabetes.

If you or someone you know has diabetes, make sure you pre-order this book, **Your D.I.A.B.E.T.E.S. Matters™** *How to Combat the Complications of Diabetes*

But I don't take sugar

It is very important that we maintain healthy levels of blood sugar. There is a huge amount of coverage in the media about how sugar is more addictive than heroin. What we do know is that sugar causes inflammation and is the major factor in weight gain/obesity and associated diseases.

When I first discovered the principles I am covering in this next section, it was a bit of a light bulb moment for me and I hope it is for you too. When I talk about sugar with my clients, particularly those that are motivated to getting healthy or losing weight, their intake of obvious sugar sources is often low and they are confused as to why they may be struggling.

One of the biggest issues is the hidden sugars in our common foods and drinks. Here is an example that may be familiar to you.

The Heart of a Woman
How to look after the heart you give to the world - Gill Barham
pg. 107

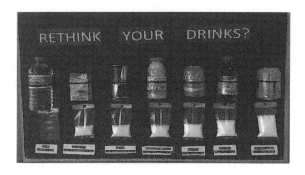

When my children were little I fell into the trap, like most parents do, thinking that my children needed a healthy breakfast of cereal or toast. I vividly remember their energy levels going up and struggling to get them all out of the door at once!

I used to teach music part-time at the local primary school and I vividly remember arriving at about 10am by which time many children were already a little lack-lustre! You may be the same? Do you grab for the coffee mid-morning to give you a boost?

Take a look at the blood sugar chart below. The chart below shows the typical fluctuations in blood sugar with our modern day diet.

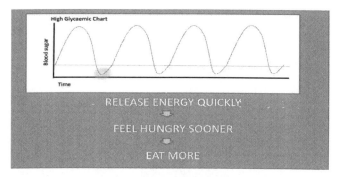

The Heart of a Woman
How to look after the heart you give to the world - Gill Barham

What do you start your day with? Your cereal may well contain high levels of sugar!! Especially if it contains dried fruits. Your bread/toast/pastry acts exactly like sugar when you eat it too and spikes your blood sugar to a dangerous level. This is actually quite dangerous for you, so your body is very efficient and produces a hormone called insulin in order to bring that blood sugar level down. Unfortunately, it's not quite as clever as we want it to be because very often that blood sugar level falls below the optimum level. Your body is even more confused now though because having a very low blood sugar is even more concerning. So it sends messages to the brain to tell you that you need to eat! So depending on a) whether you eat or b) what you eat first in a day, by mid-morning or mid-afternoon your energy levels are low and very often it's at this point that you choose foods that give you an instant boost. (That includes the sweet, chocolate, biscuit, sandwich, pastry, pasta salad or high sugar fruit snack or drink.)

When I work with my clients who want to lose weight, they are often so embarrassed because they feel under pressure that they should be able to practise "self-control" but it is this imbalance in blood sugar that is causing that lack of control over their appetite, and there is little they can do until we set their microbiome in order and then teach the basics of low GI/GL eating.

It's not your fault.

You may have been on a diet or know someone that has been on a diet or many diets, like me!! The diet industry is HUGE! The CEO of one of the most popular weekly slimming clubs has admitted that

The Heart of a Woman
How to look after the heart you give to the world - Gill Barham
pg. 109

their model is set up to fail. It is all too common for dieters to lose weight but to put that weight back on (and perhaps a little more) and then renew their subscription.

If diets worked then there would be no need for diet clubs.

www.theLifestyleLeader.co.uk

So you may be aware of the frustration and confusion over what to eat, when to eat and how much to eat to maintain a healthy weight. On The **Your H.E.A.R.T. Matters™** Programme, my clients are supplied with charts that list the most common foods and how they are broken down into sugars i.e. energy, in the body. The principle of eating food that goes into the blood stream more slowly, or by combining foods for this effect, reduces imbalances so that you can

- be more in control of what you eat
- make better healthier choices
- reduce portions naturally
- enjoy more sustained energy levels through the day

The Heart of a Woman
How to look after the heart you give to the world - Gill Barham
pg. 110

- stop cravings
- manage your weight
- avoid insulin resistance leading to type II diabetes
- control or even reverse diabetes
- improve mood

GI/GL

Let's talk about GI- glycemic index (the amount of sugar in a food) and GL - glycemic load (the speed of release into the bloodstream of that food as energy) in more detail. These two values are placed on everything we eat. In order to balance blood sugar levels, we need to limit or avoid the high glycemic index foods: those with a rating of over 70 and instead choose foods that have a rating of 55 or less. We are best to avoid or limit foods in the high GL - glycemic load category: foods rated over 15 and choose ones that are below 10.

We do need "sugar" in our system because it is our energy source for all bodily functions. This sugar from simple and complex carbohydrates is transported through the bloodstream to the liver where it is converted from glucose to glycogen. When we have too much glucose in the system that's when we land in trouble as excess glycogen is stored as fat. The slower we can make the "sugar" in your food get into your system the more likely you are to be able to control blood sugar and therefore reduce fat.

By eating slower release, low GI/GL foods, your blood sugar will be much more stable. The chart below shows a much more stable and balanced blood sugar picture.

The Heart of a Woman
How to look after the heart you give to the world - Gill Barham
pg. 111

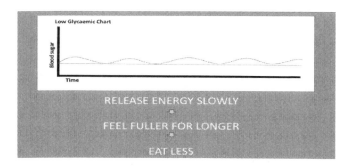

In The **Your H.E.A.R.T. Matters™** Programme we teach you how you can combine foods too to good effect by tweaking your daily habits by making some simple better choices:

BETTER CHOICES

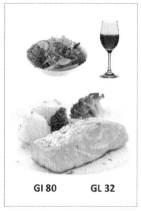

GI 80   GL 32

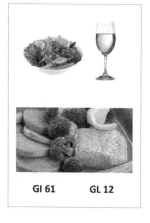

GI 61   GL 12

Salmon, new potato, broccoli, mixed salad, red wine

Salmon, sweet potato, broccoli, mixed salad, white wine.

The Heart of a Woman
How to look after the heart you give to the world - Gill Barham
pg. 112

VI.2 Balancing Hormones

The State of Female Health

You will already have a real understanding from previous chapters of some general principles in achieving good health. In this section we look specifically at women's health at all stages. When you work with me you will be able to pin point what is most relevant to you. But first let's look at some facts:

- 70% of the population is lacking in trace minerals, especially magnesium, and 1 in 5 people in the UK are deficient in vitamin D
- Infertility is increasing – 1 in 8 couples have difficulty in conceiving
- Up to 80% of women suffer with monthly PMS
- 16% of UK women report missing one or more days' work per month due to female related problems.

Hormones are the most important chemicals in the body

- Hormones give instructions to the cells in the body
- Steroid hormones such as Oestrogen, Progesterone and Testosterone require *Essential Fats* for production
- Protein-like hormones such as Insulin, HGH Thyroxin need *Complete Proteins* for production.
- ALL require a healthy LIVER.

The Heart of a Woman
How to look after the heart you give to the world - Gill Barham
pg. 113

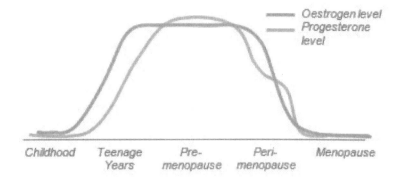

Oestrogen level
Progesterone level

Childhood   Teenage   Pre-   Peri-   Menopause
             Years   menopause   menopause

The Hormone Cycle

In second part of **The Total Body Blueprint™** we look at the stages of a woman's natural fluctuations in sex hormone levels.

Young adult

- Progesterone and Oestrogen are approaching their peak levels of production each month
- Metabolism and Fat Burning should be at its highest
- The monthly cycle should be consistent and regular

However,......

- This age group is not consuming enough protein
- Neurotransmitter production is affected, namely
  o Serotonin and
  o Melatonin production
- Anti–depressant prescriptions are currently at an all-time high for teenagers. When anti- depressants are prescribed there can be long term intestinal issues that in turn negatively impact hormone balance.

The Heart of a Woman
How to look after the heart you give to the world - Gill Barham
pg. 114

The Fertile Years
- Progesterone and Oestrogen are at their peak levels
- The Liver needs to be healthy for steroid hormone production
- Your monthly cycle should be consistent and regular
- Xenoestrogens (see chapter IV) are impacting oestrogen and testosterone balance – leading to Endometriosis, PCOS, (Poly Cystic Ovary Syndrome) PMS (Pre-Menstrual Syndrome)

Nutrition for Fertility

I know from my own experience that pre-conception and conceptual care is vital to give your baby the best of starts in life.

Remember my son Matt?

Matt is my second child and the only boy!! What a difficult place to be... the middle child with 2 strong willed sisters!

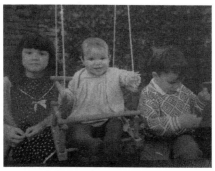

The Heart of a Woman
How to look after the heart you give to the world - Gill Barham

I am very fortunate in that I found conceiving exceptionally easy. I had a plan for how far apart I wanted my children to be in age and there wasn't anything that could alter that.

If you were with me in 1991 though, you would have seen me struggling with severe tiredness and repeated sore throats. My GP, the handsome bearded Dr P phoned with the results of my latest blood test. "Well, sorry Gill, this time the test was positive, you have glandular fever. There is nothing we can do to help, you need to rest as much as possible and perhaps try some alternate therapies".

I spent many weeks lying on the sofa trying to recover. Apart from feeling awful, I had a booking in my singing diary to sing the soprano solo in the Brahms Requiem for a local choral society concert. This was one of the many moments in my life where I really missed my Mum. She would have been with me like a shot I know, but I had no one to help out apart from my husband, who was at work all day. I remember feeling very upset whenever my fellow mums from our mother and baby group moaned about their own mothers "interfering", I could have done with some serious interference at that moment! Not for the first time, it made me think of how I took her for granted when she was alive.

What Would I Say to the 18-Year-old Me?

This question was posed by my friend and mentor, Cheryl Chapman, I thought to myself "here we go, another soul searching moment coming up in the quest for personal growth and fulfilment"

Will I be catapulted back to a time of angst, insecurity, indecision, and financial difficulties? Will I find myself giving the teenage me a

The Heart of a Woman
How to look after the heart you give to the world - Gill Barham
pg. 116

bit of a talking too? A shoulder to cry on? An encouraging hug?

Hell no!! (Sorry, bit American)

At eighteen, I felt free, totally free. I had just started a music degree at the University of East Anglia, I was studying, singing, and playing music, acting in the drama society plays, living in halls, meeting new people, and drinking too much Guinness. I had a full grant (showing my age), and a well-paid job at the weekends, so I don't recall ever having to worry about money. I had my first real date; I was asked out to dinner at Tattlers Restaurant in Pottergate, Norwich, and fell in love with Cote du Rhone! Oh and the young man who I dated for a year or so, Douglas, he played the cello and fretless bass guitar and looked a bit like Brian Cox - the scientist off the TV.

I was virtually at the other end of the country from my parents, having been brought up in Devon, and was relieved to be away from my grumpy, controlling Dad, who made our home-life one of uncertainty and anxiety because of his changing moods. I was the first of over 60 cousins to go to university, but what seemed alien to my family, just seemed like a normal and natural path for me.

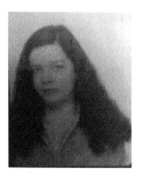

The Heart of a Woman
How to look after the heart you give to the world - Gill Barham

I wore ponchos, sandals, Laura Ashley clothes, and drank Earl Grey tea (my Mum used to get the two mixed up), shopped for local produce on Norwich Market, and owned my first ever bicycle, which I called Beryl. (Norwich is flatter than Devon).

So is here anything I would say to the young Miss Wells? Yes, phone your Mum!! At least every week! AHHH hindsight is a wonderful thing isn't it?

Sadly, although I escaped from the oppressive household, as you know, my Mum chose not to. There were obvious good times in my parents' relationship but in the end, in fact within just 10 years, she died due to the depression and illnesses she had suffered as a result of an undiagnosed reactive depression from when her own mother died and the many years of stress and unhappiness. So perhaps you can understand that my drive and purpose now is to do all I can to reduce my own risks of suffering a similar early death; (I am so like my mum) by changing the career path that was the source of my stress; learning to nourish my heart, with good habits, good people and a passion for saving lives. I am so fortunate though, in that unlike my mother, I have the best friend and partnership with my husband Peter, who I have been with for 34 years.

When I felt the acute loss of my eldest daughter leave home when she was 18, (I was a complete wreck for weeks!!) I finally understood the pain my lovely Mum must have gone through as I waltzed off into my new life at the same age. I rang home once a week - well I did in the early days, and sent the occasional letter.

Each successive child leaving home has got easier....

The Heart of a Woman
How to look after the heart you give to the world - Gill Barham
pg. 118

And now, my youngest daughter is at university in Durham, where she is studying English (and partying). In her first year she became a member of the Ultimate Frisbee society, the Pool society and the Scottish Dancing society! She wears the poncho I knitted for her, has pink sandals, retro Laura Ashley clothes, drinks Earl Grey tea, shops at her local veg market and owns her first bicycle, which she calls Violet!

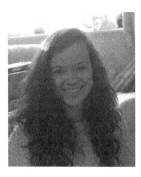

The great thing is though... We talk on FaceTime, Skype, send pictures via WhatsApp, and Facebook and all 3 children, now in their 20's, ring home on Sunday's for a chat with us both.

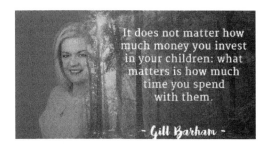

It does not matter how much money you invest in your children: what matters is how much time you spend with them.

~ Gill Barham ~

The Heart of a Woman
How to look after the heart you give to the world - Gill Barham

So back to 1991 and the Glandular fever.

To speed up my recovery, I took my GP's advice and looked to Shiatsu and Homeopathy for help. It was my first real exposure to natural forms of treatment and the first time I looked at how my diet may improve my health. These complimentary therapies did indeed help, and within a few weeks I began to feel much better. When I expressed my intention to fall pregnant, both therapists recommended that I wait a few more months. Well, that wouldn't have suited my plan would it? So within a short while I fell pregnant with Matthew. It was a very difficult pregnancy, he was 18 days early and weighed 10lbs 3oz. He started his life on the highest part of the centile chart but by 5 months old was on the lower end. He was almost a "failure to thrive" baby even though I fed him myself. He had a virus that caused similar symptoms to water on the brain, reflux, he didn't digest his food well, and had very floppy limbs. We had no diagnosis from the paediatrician, but instead took him home and worked on his motor skills and nutrition. He did begin to recover and met all of milestones, albeit he walked a little later than the girls at 16 months.

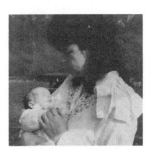

Matthew at 6 weeks old, still not back to his birth weight.

The Heart of a Woman
How to look after the heart you give to the world - Gill Barham
pg. 120

Many years later if you were with me I was at an event where I was recounting this story to a room full of therapists and health professionals. One lady, who I have subsequently been mistaken for as we look similar, came up to me at the end. "Gill, I think your son's poor start in life and his IBS diagnosis at 11 has something to do with your glandular fever. The virus causes adrenal stress and it is likely that your body will have been using Matthew's adrenals when he was in utero."

Well, it does seem likely doesn't it? It is so obvious to me now that any mother's health will have an impact on her unborn baby. Increasingly, we know to be careful about what we eat and what to avoid when pregnant or breastfeeding. Twenty five years ago, obstetricians and midwives were unconvinced about the importance of folic acid in pregnancy. The focus on the impact of a deficiency in Vit D in the medical profession is only very recent in comparison. I believe that the more work that is done in terms of the addition of vitamins, minerals and nutraceuticals on the impact of Elite Health is the way that we will combat the illness epidemics of today such as heart disease.

So prior to conception a gentle detox is a great idea because a sluggish liver and an imbalance in the microbiome compromises hormone balance and can lead to morning sickness. A detox also helps to clear Xenoestrogens.

A daily boost of Antioxidants – e.g. dark fruits and green leafy veg, helps to reduce inflammation and reduce cortisol levels.

The Heart of a Woman
How to look after the heart you give to the world - Gill Barham
pg. 121

Omega 3 fats such as pumpkin and flax seeds, oily fish, are needed for brain and membrane development, a lack can lead to post-natal depression.

Add Probiotics via a supplement and include natural yoghurt as this is important for immunity, intestinal function and further hormone balance.

The body requires high levels of Multi–vitamins and minerals especially at this stage so eat plenty of raw or lightly steamed veg, and add a safe supplement which contains a safe form of vitamin A.

A lack of vitamin B1, B2, B6 folic acid, zinc, calcium, magnesium – all have an impact on birth abnormalities

Some tips on Nutrition for Pregnancy

Weight gain in pregnancy should be around 12kgs
Less than adequate nutrition and a sluggish liver can lead to morning sickness.
Sugary foods can lead to bladder infections.
Gums may bleed due to increased oestrogen levels
Bowel movements may be impaired – so lots of fibre is needed.
Keep up your probiotics to help your baby develop a strong immune system.

Late 30" s – oh here we go - Hormone Imbalances

The Heart of a Woman
How to look after the heart you give to the world - Gill Barham
pg. 122

In **The Total Body Blueprint™** we look in more detail at the types of PMS that you may be experiencing. It is important to note that most hormonal problems for younger women and girls are linked to the similar triggers experienced in the Perimenopause. It is therefore important to recognise that Endometriosis, Polycystic Ovary Syndrome, Infertility, and PMS can be linked to a more troublesome menopausal journey and are all managed in similar ways depending on each individual needs.

Are you ready for the menopause?

Studies show that women in the UK can experience menopausal symptoms for up to 14 years, and If you are in your early to mid-40s - You MAY already be in the Perimenopause phase....

Not sure?   Do any of these sound familiar?

- Menstrual Problems
- PMS,
- Paranoia
- Irritation
- Panic
- Pre-menstrual and menstrual migraine
- Insomnia, tiredness
- Joint aches
- Flu like symptoms
- Poor concentration, verbal memory
- Loss of Libido, loos of drive
- Inability to multitask
- Inability to cope

The Heart of a Woman
How to look after the heart you give to the world - Gill Barham
pg. 123

You may already be experiencing some or all if these symptoms without realising that it MAY be your hormones putting you out of whack!

You may even feel you are going slightly bonkers!

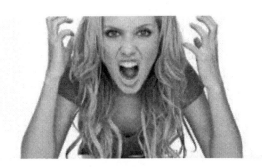

Depending on the stage of this process, my clients regularly report such feelings as:

- *I would like to KNOW if I am menopausal but can't tell and I've heard that GP tests aren't that helpful.*

- *I want to avoid conventional medications such as HRT, but can't work out where to go for help*

- *I am feeling a bit frustrated and anxious for the future and see no clear pathway to being as happy, desirable and fulfilled as I was in my 30's or 40's.*

The Heart of a Woman
How to look after the heart you give to the world - Gill Barham
pg. 124

- *I'm finding it difficult to put myself first and increasingly focus more on those around me as I have both teenagers and elderly parents.*

- *I don't want to look and feel old! I'm beginning to feel that I am losing my identity as a woman, feel invisible at times and I am mourning the younger me.*

- *I have given up; have taken to the biscuit barrel and the sofa thinking because there is no hope for me! (I feel like hiding away)*

- *I am focusing on what hasn't worked already and why I am likely to fail again.*

- *I see other ladies coping well with this phase in their life and I'm wondering how they do it!*

- *I am finding it all a bit overwhelming especially as I am juggling family and work life and sometimes I'm pretty exhausted!*

- *I am safely through the other side but I am worried about keeping my bones and heart healthy.*

If any of these ring true for you, then stay with me.

I'm going to give you some valuable information to help you to feel confident and knowledgeable about:

The Heart of a Woman
How to look after the heart you give to the world - Gill Barham

1. What the menopause is,
2. What you need to eat,
3. What you need to avoid,
4. What else you need to do nutritionally to SAIL through this natural process

.... So that you can relax, stop worrying and take control of the next rewarding phase of your life.

"And the beauty of a woman, with passing years only grows"
Audrey Hepburn,
Actress

Knowledge is power....

The Heart of a Woman
How to look after the heart you give to the world - Gill Barham
pg. 126

WARNING. .... This is NOT for you though if....

1. You are the person who relies on conventional treatments and medications only.
2. You are closed to the hard facts about our modern day nutritional state and how it is affecting your health.
3. You want conclusive evidence that making small changes will work for you before you will even try something new.
4. You are not willing to invest in your own health and put yourself first.

However, ... If you are ready to get to some **simple** facts, some **great advice** and strategies for a healthier, happier and wonderfully feminine you... Then keep reading!

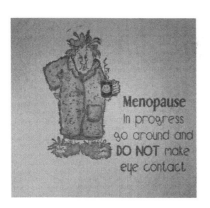

The Heart of a Woman
How to look after the heart you give to the world - Gill Barham

<u>The 3 phases of the **Menopause**</u>

The Menopause isn't a disease – although the standard response from the medical profession and drugs companies is to "treat" the symptoms with medications. Your GP will very often only have HRT to offer you, but hopefully you will appreciate after reading this, that this may not be your best option

The Menopause itself is actually the last day of your periods. However, it's never possible to know that! Studies show currently that the average age of the LAST day of a woman's periods in the UK is 51.

So the Perimenopause, which can last up to 10 years, is where the symptoms start to appear.
Let's look at the two that often cause the most distress: The vasomotor symptoms of hot flushes and night sweats. These are caused by dilation of the blood vessels and increased flow of blood to the head and neck, causing reddening of the skin and sweating.

In a study reported in JAMA Internal Medicine researchers in the US looked at 1,449 women from 1996 - 2013 with frequent hot flushes or night sweats. It is the largest study of its kind and included four ethnic groups. Here's what they found:
- The average length of time women endured symptoms was 7.4 years.
- Half of the women were affected for less than that time, but half had symptoms longer — some for at least 14 years.
- African-American women experience symptoms for the longest amount of time, an average of 10.1 years, while

The Heart of a Woman
How to look after the heart you give to the world - Gill Barham
pg. 128

Japanese women had symptoms for 4.8 years. (In fact, there is no actual word for the menopause in Japan! - more on that later.)

The study's lead author, Professor Nancy Avis, said *'The duration of 7.4 years highlights the limitations of guidance recommending short-term hormone therapy and emphasises the need to identify safe long-term therapies for the treatment of vasomotor symptoms.'*

Dr JoAnn E. Manson, chief of preventive medicine at the Harvard-affiliated Brigham and Women's Hospital and an author of a commentary on the study, said *'Women with more stress in their lives may be more aware of their symptoms and perceive them to be more bothersome."*

'But also having significant night sweats that interrupt sleep can lead to stress' she added.

Apart from those already mentioned, symptoms may include:
Mood swings
Bloating
Anxiety
Heart Palpitations
Headaches
Lack of energy/ Reduced stamina

It is also very common to experience:
Depression
Poor self-esteem / Low self-image.

The Heart of a Woman
How to look after the heart you give to the world - Gill Barham
pg. 129

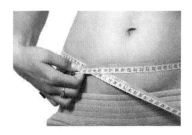

And to start putting on **WEIGHT**,

.........very often around the middle.

During this phase and also postmenopausal, you may also see changes such as:

- Vaginal dryness
- Dry, Aging skin

Studies have found that women with hot flush symptoms also face increased risk of cardiovascular problems and bone loss. So the big concern as hormone levels decline is to avoid Osteoporosis and Heart Attack or Stroke.

WE HAVE A CHOICE.

Wait for illness to happen OR Begin living well today!

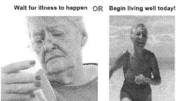

These two women are approximately the same age.

The Heart of a Woman
How to look after the heart you give to the world - Gill Barham

NOTE: many of these symptoms listed can also be attributed to other things. So it would be wrong to automatically assume that just because you're of a certain age 'it must be the menopause".

You could be suffering from
- *Blood sugar or other hormonal imbalances,*
- *Nutrient deficiencies*
- *Poor liver function,*
- *Essential fatty acid depletion*
- *Adrenal stress (it is quite common for the 2 to be confused and you may be prescribed HRT for this!)*

So what's actually going on? (The science bit)

Normally, during a woman's monthly cycle, oestrogen is released after a period in order to stimulate production of an egg, and the build-up of a rich lining to the womb. At around the time of ovulation the production of oestrogen peaks and then tails off. If an egg is produced the empty egg sac, called the corpus luteum, starts to produce progesterone and this is the more dominant of the two hormones for the latter half of the cycle.

During the perimenopause, (usually early to late-40s) an egg isn't produced every month.

If an egg isn't produced then there is no corpus luteum, and no progesterone. So often some of the effects a woman feels are down to too little progesterone, or what is called **oestrogen dominance**

The Heart of a Woman
How to look after the heart you give to the world - Gill Barham
pg. 131

(much of the medical approach i.e. HRT, is to put in more oestrogen, rather than trying to balance existing levels)

So successfully dealing with the menopause is about **maintaining** hormone balance as these levels naturally start to tail of.

Artificially maintaining these levels is really not the best answer to dealing with this life stage, as nature intends for them to be reduced. (This is what HRT or other unregulated Bioidentical "natural" hormone therapy does.)

Each woman's response to the menopause is going to be individual depending on what else is going on in her body.

Hormone levels are influenced by:
1. Ethnicity
2. The natural, gradual decline in production of both of these hormones by the ovaries
3. Stress - extra oestrogen is usually produced from the adrenals – but this is diminished by the stress hormone, Cortisol.
4. Artificial lowered levels of Cholesterol (statin use) can also have a negative impact.
5. A poor functioning gut, liver and intestines (elimination and detoxification system), means that hormones are not excreted effectively, and keep circulating to cause imbalance.
6. Exposure to Xenoestrogens: these can be thought of as false oestrogens, which also contribute to oestrogen dominance.

The Heart of a Woman
How to look after the heart you give to the world - Gill Barham
pg. 132

For more information on these endocrine disruptors please revisit
Chapter V.

So, what can YOU do to help?

Let's look at some FACTS AND MYTHS about HRT

HRT helps you to avoid the menopause – NO in most cases, HRT merely delays the process and whether you are taking it for 2, 5 or 10 years, you are likely to still experience the symptoms of the menopause that you had when you started taking it. I speak from personal experience here, having had a hysterectomy at 45 and like many women was given HRT as I was under 50 years of age, regardless of the fact that I still have my ovaries. My perimenopausal symptoms started up when I decided that the risks associated with HRT out-weighed the benefits and stopped the patches and I still have to be really on top of my symptoms which I believe were not helped by many decades on the contraceptive pill.

We are back to our hindsight again!!

HRT is safe to take – It is important to note that too much oestrogen can lead to cancerous growths in both the breast and womb. So the right balance is vital – this is where HRT becomes a problem, as it keeps oestrogen levels un-naturally high, in comparison to progesterone, therefore raising the risk of breast and ovarian cancer.

HRT will keep me healthy and looking younger for longer. Well yes and no, because of the increased risks. The best way to move into

The Heart of a Woman
How to look after the heart you give to the world - Gill Barham
pg. 133

the next phase of your hormonal life is to nourish the body so that it can balance and stabilise the effects of the natural drop in hormones and provide high levels of nutrients that are targeted at anti-ageing.

HRT is the best way to avoid Osteoporosis – although a decrease in oestrogen affects your risk of bone weakness, HRT is not the safest way to improve your bone density.

HRT keeps me safe from heart disease. ......

When you work with me you will learn the best way to support your bones, your heart, how to keep yourself looking a feeling younger with targeted supplementation and nutraceuticals that fill the gaps that we have talked about in chapter V.

In the meantime, here's what you can do naturally with food

Let's look at your Diet.

1. Phytoestrogens can help reduce hot flushes and night sweats – so eat lots of pulses such as lentils, chickpeas and (good quality, non GMO) soy. (The low levels of oestrogen in Japanese women is attributed to the consumption of soy)
2. Garlic is also good, as are seeds such as linseeds, pumpkin seeds, sesame etc.
3. Include whole grains such a brown rice, barley, oats and rye,
4. Lots of vegetables, especially the green leafy ones,
5. Fruit

The Heart of a Woman
How to look after the heart you give to the world - Gill Barham
pg. 134

6. Herbs and spices such as cinnamon, sage, red clover, fennel and parsley.
7. Sprouts such as mung beans and alfalfa.
8. Oily fish and nuts and seeds like Chia can help increase your intake of the beneficial Omega oils.
9. Fibre is essential to regulate bowel action. This can help prevent bloating and flatulence, help prevent disease, lower cholesterol and help carry toxins out of the body. (Many of us struggle to get enough fibre, particularly the soluble variety into our diets, so fibre supplements are vital).

Cut back on tea, coffee, fizzy drinks, squashes and alcohol which can dehydrate; because blood sugar (therefore mood) swings, contribute to hormonal imbalance, and weight gain.

10. Drink plenty of water, as the less you drink the more your body will hold onto what you do take in. Often the response to water retention is to cut down on the amount of fluid taken in, which can just make matters worse. Drink FILTERED rather than tap or bottled water.

Now what you should avoid:

1. Processed foods: (anything 'white' i.e. sugar, flour, bread etc.), convenience foods and stimulants such as caffeine, which all cause:
• blood sugar swings,
• contribute to irritability,
• moodiness,
• sweating,
• forgetfulness,

The Heart of a Woman
How to look after the heart you give to the world - Gill Barham
pg. 135

- depression and
- tiredness,

2. Artificial sweeteners such as aspartame (NutraSweet) are NOT GOOD FOR YOU, so avoid them at all costs – this includes diet drinks and 'sugar-free' drinks & foods.
3. Red meat and dairy produce should be cut back on. They are high in saturated fats and have an acidifying action on the body. (Lemon water and Alkaline drinks help to alkalise the body)
4. Additives, high salt diets (use Himalayan or natural salts) and GM foods.
5. Statins that bring your cholesterol levels down to beyond a healthy range. Good cholesterol is required for the production of the steroid hormones, oestrogen, progesterone and testosterone.

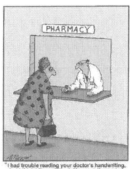

"I had trouble reading your doctor's handwriting, but I think I figured it out. However, if you start to drool uncontrollably or gain more than 15 pounds in a week, stop taking them."

A word about exercise for this period in your life.

The Heart of a Woman
How to look after the heart you give to the world - Gill Barham
pg. 136

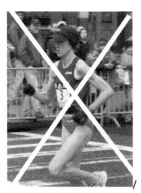

Undertake some **short burst exercise** programme or do some walking, swimming, Yoga or Pilates. Gentle weight bearing exercises are good for maintaining bone density and strength.

Cardio exercises like running, even on a treadmill is **stressful** for the body, so avoid these, even if you are used to it. It will produce more free radical damage and speed up the ageing process.

Of course, it is your choice, but the fitness experts that I work with all agree that we should modify our type of exercise as we age.

As part of The **Your H.E.A.R.T. Matters™** Programme we discuss the best forms of exercise for you.

The Heart of a Woman
How to look after the heart you give to the world - Gill Barham
pg. 137

VI.3 Building Health

The past few years for me have been about understanding the difference between treating symptoms and building health. As a nurse, I was trained to look at disease processes and symptomatic relief. Whilst I am a big fan of conventional medicine in its right place, I am much more interested in the effect that living a healthy lifestyle can have on longevity and wellness. Whatever complimentary therapies you enjoy, for example: Essential oils, Reiki, Shiatsu, Acupuncture, Bowen Therapy, Colour Therapy, Mindfulness, EFT, and I have used most of them at one time or another, I believe that the root of Elite Health is what you are putting in your mouth!

Our western diet is calorie dense but nutrient deficient.

In my experience, when you are trying to get well, stay well or overcome illness, although food choices are vitally important, there is increasing evidence that the many gaps in our everyday nutrition that are instrumental to the decline of the nation's health and contribute to the lifestyle diseases we see more of today such as:

- Obesity (1/3 of the adult population)
- Diabetes - type 2 (rates set to double again in the next 5 years)
- Thyroid issues

The Heart of a Woman
How to look after the heart you give to the world - Gill Barham
pg. 138

- Auto immune diseases such as ME/ chronic fatigue /Fibromyalgia
- Arthritis/osteoporosis
- IBS
- Hormone imbalances such as PCOS, endometriosis, PMS, moobs, (man boobs) and symptoms of the menopause!

I could go on!

Anyone who smokes, is on medication of any kind or has stress in their lives, is even more vulnerable to nutritional deficiency. Ethnicity also impacts your particular nutritional requirements.

Five a day

Do you recall section 3 of The **Essential Energy Elevator**™? How did you do? Do you get the daily nutrients you need?

Let's look at why you may need to fill the gaps in your diet:

The Heart of a Woman
How to look after the heart you give to the world - Gill Barham
pg. 139

WELLNESS Questionnaire

The questions below are designed to give you a complete overview of how you are feeling right now and a way to track your progress over the next 90 days.

Please score each question using the words in CAPITAL LETTERS for each section. Some answers require a number. **If a question is not relevant for you, please enter N/A**

Alert:
Start the scoring in the right-hand column. This way you are able to fold the paper and hide your first scores when you complete the second and third months.

Add any other concerns/conditions you have in the blank spaces provided or add more below.

Several conditions have room for you to enter the locations in the body. Against "swelling", you could write;" left ankle", for example.

Please be as accurate as you can as this will help you monitor how you feel – for example, we often don't know we've been out of pain until we are back in it! So, even if you don't have a problem with your hair, still give it a score as you may notice an improvement!

Everyone has the right to Elite Health.

The Heart of a Woman
How to look after the heart you give to the world - Gill Barham
pg. 140

General health	Month 3	Month 2	Month 1
ENTER GREAT, FAIR OR POOR			
Hair quality			
Hair quantity			
Skin			
Eyesight with glasses			
Eyesight without glasses			
Hearing			
Energy level - morning			
Energy level - midday			
Energy level - afternoon			
Energy level - evening			
Sleep - quantity			
Sleep - quality			
Alertness on waking			
Brittle finger nails			
Mental alertness			
Memory			
General mood			
General stiffness			
General mobility			
General flexibility			
Muscle strength			
Overall feeling of wellbeing			
Happiness			
Stress levels			
Ease of going back to sleep			

The Heart of a Woman
How to look after the heart you give to the world - Gill Barham
pg. 141

Times getting up in the night NUMBER			
Sleep - NUMBER of hours			

START HERE

Aches and pains LOCATION SEVERE, MODERATE MILD OR N/A IF RELEVANT	Month 3	Month 2	Month 1
Headaches - severity			
Headaches – number			
Migraines - number			
Neck			
Shoulder(s)			
Arms e.g. R forearm			
Elbows			
Wrists			
Hands			
Fingers			
Upper back			
Mid back			
Lower back			
Hips			
Knees			
Ankles			
Feet			
Legs			
Stomach			
Teeth/gums			

The Heart of a Woman
How to look after the heart you give to the world - Gill Barham

pg. 142

Mouth ulcers			
Sinuses			
Itchy skin -			
Pins and needles - e.g. fingers			
Numbness -			
Swelling -			

START HERE

Digestion ENTER FREQENTLY OCCASIONALY OR NEVER	Month 3	Month 2	Month 1
Nausea			
Acid reflux			
Bloating			
Abdominal cramp/wind			
BOWELS – (what' s normal for you)	x	x	x
Frequency e.g. 1 x a day, 3 x day, 3 x a week			
Constipation			
Diarrhoea			
ENTER SEVERE, MODERATE OR MILD			
Appetite			
Cravings			
Food sensitivities/allergies			

The Heart of a Woman
How to look after the heart you give to the world - Gill Barham

PMT/Menopause ENTER SEVERE, MODERATE MILD or N/A	Month 3	Month 2	Month 1
Painful periods			
Heavy periods			
Breast tenderness			
Bloating			
Headaches			
PCOS			
Endometriosis			
Moodiness/irritability			
Hot flushes (number in day)			
Hot flushes (severity - day)			
Hot flushes (number in night)			
Hot flushes (severity - night)			
Itchy skin -			
Anxiety/panic attacks			
Paranoia			
Irritation			
Insomnia			
Loss of libido			
Inability to cope			
Poor concentration/verbal memory			
Joint aches			
Regularity (cycle)			
Colour of blood Bright or dark red			
Clots ENTER SEVERE, MODERATE MILD or N/A			

The Heart of a Woman
How to look after the heart you give to the world - Gill Barham
pg. 144

My other symptoms:

Please also add your own ENTER SEVERE, MODERATE MILD or N/A	Month 3	Month 2	Month 1
Blood sugar levels (average reading)			
Thyroxine results (average reading)			
Weight			
Cholesterol level Number			
Blood pressure (average reading)			
Bladder (leaking, cystitis etc)			
Lungs/breathing			
Yeast/fungal infections			
Mucous/congestion			
Dizziness			
Exercise Ave number of sessions per week and/or Ave number of steps per day			

So the conventional approach may be to wait for the flashing lights that you have identified here to force you to take action, visit your GP, possibly receive a diagnosis and be prescribed some therapy or more often medication. Or, when you work with me, you will learn more about a more preventative approach, how to perfect your personal nutrition and fitness regime to achieve Elite Health.

Once you have your personalised plan, you can use this chart to monitor your progress.

Good health is all about creating good habits
The Heart of a Woman
How to look after the heart you give to the world - Gill Barham

You will see a gradual improvement in your answers as your body is helped back into a balanced state. You can expect to enjoy a greater sense of wellbeing if you stick to your recommendations. With this programme the small changes you are going to make are easy to maintain and therefore more effective long term.

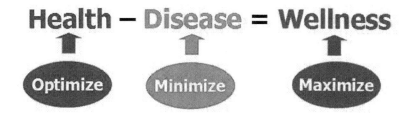

The Heart of a Woman
How to look after the heart you give to the world - Gill Barham
pg. 146

"We Need to Stop Treating Disease and Start Building Good Health"

Steven Horne

The Heart of a Woman
How to look after the heart you give to the world - Gill Barham
pg. 147

I love food

I am very proud that all of my children, now all in their 20's, cook their food from fresh and enjoy eating a healthy diet. Even though they have super busy lives, they all appreciate the benefits of reducing their exposure to processed foods, and shop where they can for local produce. I seem to have successfully instilled an 80/20 rule – one that is manageable and allows for fun and flexibility. (Eat healthily for 80% and allow for some less healthy foods and beverages!! 20% of the time). This diagram, based on the Julie Danulik food pyramid give you an idea of the proportions of the nutrients you need daily.

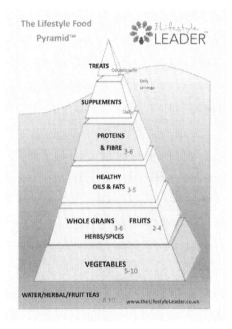

The Heart of a Woman
How to look after the heart you give to the world - Gill Barham

"Let food be thy medicine, let medicine be thy food." Albert Einstein.

But is that enough?

Well in my opinion, sadly not. With all the knowledge I have gained and the results I have witnessed from my clients, I am totally convinced that the majority of the population need to add good, natural, tested, quality supplementation into a daily regime. You will see the addition of supplementation at the top of the pyramid.

At the very least, you may be aware that one of the key vitamins that we are deficient in, very commonly in the UK, is Vitamin D3. GP's are testing for deficiency nowadays and even prescribing (an inferior) supplement for patients. We can only manufacture this

The Heart of a Woman
How to look after the heart you give to the world - Gill Barham
pg. 149

vitamin, which is actually a hormone, under the skin through exposure to sunlight. However, we require 15 mins of exposure a day without sunscreen, but the position of the sun between October to April in the UK does not allow for proper exposure. People with darker skins are particularly at risk of a deficiency. (Functional Nutritionists are aware that a simple D3 supplement is often the sole solution to prevent miscarriage in Asian women). D3 is so vital for many functions in the body, not least, heart health, bone health, intestinal function and to prevent depression, especially SAD (Seasonal Affective Disorder). This is a brief summary of findings on the positive effect of Vitamin D for Asthma sufferers:

"The researchers also found that vitamin D can help cut the rate of asthma sufferers needing steroid treatment.

The Cochrane review's lead researcher, Professor Adrian Martineau, said vitamin D "significantly reduced the risk of severe asthma attacks, without causing side effects".

He added that taking vitamin D on a regular basis reduced the risk of asthma sufferers requiring a hospital admission or a visit to A&E from 6 per cent to 3 per cent.

The researchers also found the rate of asthma attack sufferers needing steroid treatment dropped from 0.44 to 0.28 attacks per person per year.

The daily dose of vitamin D used in the study was between 25 to 50 micrograms, which is much higher than the government recommendation of 10 micrograms per day... and according to many alternative health practitioners the dosage used in the study is at the lower end of the scale when it comes to the therapeutic benefits of vitamin D."

The Heart of a Woman
How to look after the heart you give to the world - Gill Barham
pg. 150

In a similar way to folic acid, which for tens of years was poo pooed as necessary by midwives and obstetricians even, is now recommended in pregnancy and for women trying to conceive. The acceptance of the need for supplementation is very slow within the traditional medical world, largely due to the severe lack of education within their training, and the influence and domination of the Pharmaceutical industry, i.e. MONEY, on the health of our nations. I see a sea change on its way though, so keep your eyes peeled and your hearts open as we have more and more evidence of the benefits of extra nutritional boosters.

7 reasons why we need to supplement:

1. Modern day intensive farming
It was reported way back in 1996 at The World Health Summit that the mineral content of or soil has reduced by 72% over the last 100 years. There is 25% less vit C in a cauliflower, 88% less iron in watercress and other countries have similar reductions in the health of their soil too. Farmers rarely REST the land between crops these days and the use of herbicides and pesticides are responsible for the reduction of essential **microbes** in the soil. (Think of the days when you used to get little hard bugs on your car windscreen that were hard to shift? Microbes!) If there are no microbes in the soil, no minerals in our food, none in us!

2. Processed foods.
There are foods that you know are processed, such as breads, cakes, ready meals, etc. but some less obvious like the bagged salad that looks healthy! It has been washed in a 20% chlorine solution and contains NO nutrient content. My recommendation is to use foods

The Heart of a Woman
How to look after the heart you give to the world - Gill Barham
pg. 151

with only 1 ingredient... So you can make your (wholemeal) lasagne, pizza, Caesar salad or banana loaf.... Just don't buy it readymade!

3. Poor food storage methods.
It is not uncommon for our fruit and veg to be put in cold storage for up to 1 year! Foods are often sprayed with enzymes too which will affect our ability to get the goodness from them. If you can afford to eat organic, your priorities should be apples, pears, tomatoes and root veg.

4. Busy lifestyles.
It is true that for women, our lifestyles have dramatically changed over the past 40 decades. We are much busier, with the demands of a family, work and social life, and stress, whether good or bad, perceived or not perceived, is a major factor in female general health. This is because of the hormones adrenaline and cortisol. Renowned herbalist, nutritional therapist and naturopath, Steven Horne highlights that men are designed to produce these hormones to protect and serve and can also release them from their system effectively. (Work hard, play hard, rest and recover). However we ladies do not eliminate these hormones as well and so they build up in the system, causing hormonal disruption and adrenal stress.

5. Limited access to daily organic foods.
Even with the best will in the world, it may be difficult to eat nutrient dense food every day.

6. Vitamin and Mineral Depletion through over use of prescription and over the counter medications.

7. The body NEVER catches up on a "bad" day.

The Heart of a Woman
How to look after the heart you give to the world - Gill Barham
pg. 152

So, you will get much, much better results if you boost your nutrition with food state supplements. (I don't mean the synthetic stuff off the supermarket or high street shelves or what is available online, as almost NONE of these products is regularly tested for safety, purity or potency)

So I only use and recommend the highest quality food state supplements in the world that are Patented, Clinically Trialled and Quality Assured. I use a company that:

- started the process of encapsulating herbs 41 years ago!
- Employ over 50 scientists, herbalists and pharmacognacists and have devoted a floor of their facility in Utah to undertaking Clinical Trials of their formulations under the guidance of Dr Matt Tripp.
- is one of a handful of supplements companies that are not owned by a pharmaceutical and are cash rich.
- is floated on the stock market and owe no money so can afford to spend huge amounts each year to obtain the highest grade organic and wild crafted ingredients from around the world.
- is renowned and respected for testing every product and formulation with over 600 processes for the best efficacy, purity and potency. (85% of supplements on the market today are produced synthetically by manufacturers and supplied to stores who then brand with their label, these companies batch test at best).

The Heart of a Woman
How to look after the heart you give to the world - Gill Barham
pg. 153

"The most expensive supplement is the one that doesn't work" Dr Matt Tripp

So if you are going to take my recommendations, please make sure that you use only food state, organic and wild crafted nutritional boosters.

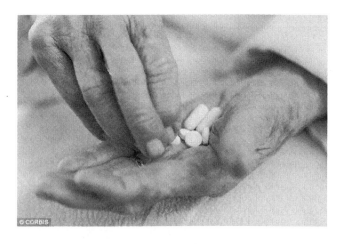

The Heart of a Woman
How to look after the heart you give to the world - Gill Barham

Let's look in more detail at just ONE of the vital minerals that we need to live a healthy life.

Magnesium...Why do we need it?

It's a mineral that is very easy for the body to lose... You can't magic magnesium!
We are at a disadvantage environmentally. As we have already covered, our soil contains less than 72% of the mineral content compared to 100 years ago and magnesium is not replenished by most growers.

Top Tip: If you grow your own veg.. You can put magnesium sulphate, (Epsom salts) on your own veggie patch.

A LACK of magnesium is implicated in so many conditions:
Circulatory
- poor circulation,
- Heart attacks,
- blood pressure issues
- sexual dysfunction
Cancer
Kidney problems
Constipation
Diabetes
Sleep issues
Migraines
Muscle pain
Bloating
Auto immune disorders such as
- ME

The Heart of a Woman
How to look after the heart you give to the world - Gill Barham
pg. 155

- Fibromyalgia

Magnesium deficiency is often misdiagnosed because it does not show up in blood tests – only 1% of the body's magnesium is stored in the blood.

So what is happening that makes magnesium so important?

This is the science bit as I understand it at a Cellular level.... we have 4 electrolytes that play a part in good health:

- Calcium & Sodium.
These two inhabit the outside of the cell for the most part.

Now if you have:
- A stressful lifestyle,
- a poor diet consisting of processed or "on the go" food, which is high in saturated fats, sugar & salt,
if you have lots of
- milk products,
- wheat based foods.
Then this body will be highly acidic. This starts changing the gut bacteria .... And compromises the ability to process and absorb nutrients
And then these factors make these 2 electrolytes over dominant.

Amongst other things, this has the effect of attracting water uptake - and extra sodium (salt) leads to bloating.

- Magnesium & Potassium inhabit the inside of the cell

Their role is to draw in lipids (fats) and clear out toxins from the cell.

The Heart of a Woman
How to look after the heart you give to the world - Gill Barham
pg. 156

At night magnesium and potassium move back into the cell to help the liver cleanse and detoxify ready for the next day.

First thing in the morning then, this is the happy situation for our cells but as the day progresses the charge in the cell is released and magnesium is lost.

In people with auto immune disease, such as Fibromyalgia and ME this movement is being hindered. Magnesium is important for energy in the cells (ATP) NSP Magnesium Malate is particularly good for ME type illnesses.

With an imbalance of these electrolytes, the cell is dehydrated or the cell is in a state of tension.
This is because Calcium and Sodium = Constriction
And Potassium and Magnesium = relaxation

This inability for the cells to relax leads to conditions such as asthma, migraines and restless legs syndrome.
We are also more prone to arthritis as Calcium is held in the joints.

Higher levels of Calcium also affect the formation of Arteriosclerosis and affects cholesterol levels.

Magnesium is key to managing constipation as we need both movements of relaxation and constriction to create peristalsis. If magnesium levels are low, there is no relaxation phase.

Magnesium also helps to keep stress hormones under control.
Stress strips the body of magnesium. Leading to Anxiety ....
Palpitations.... Weight loss.... We need magnesium to produce

The Heart of a Woman
How to look after the heart you give to the world - Gill Barham
pg. 157

Serotonin, anti-depressants such as Prozac don't replace the magnesium!

Magnesium opens up the glucose channels in the cell wall .... So without it insulin bounces off the cells. This is a factor in Insulin resistance and Polycyclic Ovary Syndrome. At the point of ovulation, magnesium levels drop. In the last 2 weeks of the menstrual cycle they are very low. Because magnesium helps to process fats if they are lacking then you can't produce Prostaglandins (the sex hormones) that balance the glandular system. Hot flushes can deplete the body of magnesium.

Suffering from PMT symptoms such as bloating and headaches is relieved by magnesium which changes the brain chemistry to establish a better electrolyte balance.

So can you take too much? Yes, you could get hypotension! But this is really only likely if on a low calcium diet. However, our food is naturally rich in Calcium and is very commonly fortified.

So.... Magnesium is more prone to loss than any other.

It is also very difficult to digest, as the cell wall, particularly if dehydrated, is hard. This is more common if you have low stomach acid and it is recommended that you take Food Enzymes to ensure effectiveness.

When you take away stress, (which creates dehydration by the way) the better you will digest your food. This is why it's important to relax when you eat. We also need to address our thoughts, our body pH and practice how to breathe.

The Heart of a Woman
How to look after the heart you give to the world - Gill Barham

Top tips:

- Take magnesium away from food.
- Drink 2 litres of water a day and add liquid chlorophyll.
- Take food enzymes.
- Reduce stress
- Look at alkalising your body with appropriate foods. (Correct breathing helps this too)

The Heart of a Woman
How to look after the heart you give to the world - Gill Barham
pg. 159

CHAPTER VII

Prosperity

This chapter is meant for you if you want to have a little more income. You may only want to be able to pay for some higher quality nutrition by generating an extra £100- £200 a month. Equally, this chapter is for you if you have bigger dreams or goals for yourself and your family.

You may be in a job or have your own business already, so I thought we might start by looking at an example of an ideal way to generate an income of whatever level you set.

A 2016 survey, featured in one our major newspapers, highlighted that the average British family have no savings. That 1 in 3 working families with children reported that if one working parent lost their job or even had a reduction in hours, they would only be able to pay their rent or mortgage for 1 month!! This leaves them feeling vulnerable and exposed to hardship. It also reported that Britain has the longest working hours in Europe and that women are the major care givers.

So it is very important to me to be able to open my clients hearts up to the possibilities, in relation to the 3rd aspect of "Wellbeing", of ways to create a more secure financial future for themselves and their loved-ones. There are, happily, a variety of opportunities in which to generate an income these days with more and more

The Heart of a Woman
How to look after the heart you give to the world - Gill Barham
pg. 160

entrepreneurship, property options and online businesses. However most require either investment, a certain amount of risk, a willingness to go it alone, or indeed all three.

Your dream job

We all have a product, a company or a business that we use and love. What if we owned a business like that? A concept we wished we had thought of, or given the chance to be part of that company?

Perhaps it is a restaurant that has the best food and atmosphere. Or better – A shop or online store with fabulous products and customer service.

I want you to imagine now that you go and speak to the MD or owner of that company or business and say: -
"I really love your business and I'm so passionate about your product, I would love to work for you. I am passionate about entrepreneurship; really ambitious and hard-working and I know I will be a success for you, but in return I would like the following: -

1. *To earn 25% commission on everything I sell.*
2. *Anything I buy for myself, I would like to buy at wholesale price.*
3. *Oh and I only want to work part time; the hours that suit me, that work around my family and other commitments.*
4. *I really enjoy working with my family and friends so would like them to be able to work here with me also.*
5. *And when someone that I introduce makes some commission on their sales, I would like you to MATCH the commission and give me the same amount as each one of them each month.*

The Heart of a Woman
How to look after the heart you give to the world - Gill Barham
pg. 161

6. *Also, when I introduce a new worker, I would expect to receive a cash bonus.*
7. *I am very ambitious and will do well, so when I do, I would like lots of recognition, achieve awards and receive all expenses paid five-star travel to countries all around the world.*
8. *I want there to be no limits to being able to advance through the company and I would like to do it at my own pace.*
9. *I really love to learn, so would require lots of free training and support and to be able to call you whenever I need your help.*
10. *Oh and when in the future I decide I don't want to be actively working the hours and perhaps want to take more holidays, I would like to still be receiving my full wages.*

Would that be OK?"

So how does that sound to you?

How does it compare to your current job business?

Would this kind of opportunity give your more time/money/freedom? Would it give you more choices? What would you do with an extra income? Would you invest it? Spend it? Give it away perhaps?

This is a true representation of what you can achieve with a Network Marketing Business (NWM) and specifically with Synergy Worldwide.

The Heart of a Woman
How to look after the heart you give to the world - Gill Barham
pg. 162

Now don't panic!!

It's possible that an MLM or NWM business model may be a new concept to you or you may be dead against it because of bad press or a previous experience. I often hear… oh isn't that pyramid selling?

Suffice to say that the world wide turnover of NWM businesses globally in 2015 was **180 Billion Dollars.** Does this suggest that they indulge in illegal or unethical practices to you?

It is clear that there are some good and many poor companies, which is the same as in any industry, so your only decision is to undertake due diligence before you commit to building a business in association with any MLM or NWM company.

My motivation for choosing to be part of a NWM company is represented by the following seven S.U.C.C.E.S.S. principles:

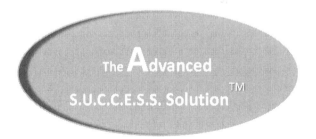

The Heart of a Woman
How to look after the heart you give to the world - Gill Barham
pg. 163

VIII.I

Support

Have you ever thought of starting your own business? Perhaps you are a business owner already or you are self-employed?

Author and entrepreneur, Robert Kyosaki illustrates the routes to financial freedom and recommends that "a *minimum* of one third of your total income should come from a source, or sources, other than your *principle* source of income."

What does your financial profile look like?

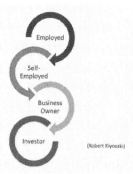

The Route to Financial Independence

With the rising numbers of unemployed in the UK and one million workers on zero contracts, there has never been a better time for starting a business from home. I saw an example recently of how difficult young families are finding life in the UK in particular. In a report written by Phillip Inman, the Economics correspondent in the Guardian Newspaper in October 2016, the UK was singled out as being among the worst countries in the developed world to be a

The Heart of a Woman
How to look after the heart you give to the world - Gill Barham
pg. 164

young mother (with a partner) seeking work. There is a definite shift and an interest in finding ways to work family life around a home-based business.

However, most businesses require considerable investment, can be risky, and often require undertaking all the roles that make a business successful, so that you end up working more hours often for less return and having less fun!

I am very conscious of this as a Pilates teacher, and working in the field of complementary therapies. A very common complaint I hear from my fellow heart-based business owners, is that they feel unsupported, isolated and alone. Even though their days are spent with clients, this is not the same as being part of a team or having colleagues with whom to share ideas and challenges.

One benefit of starting a business in Network Marketing is the unprecedented amount of support available to you, when you choose the right company and a proactive sponsor or mentor.

The great thing about having a NWM business is that you can choose your hours, the amount of income you want, the rate at which you want to achieve it and most importantly, **who** you work with and help to achieve their dreams and goals. No more Miss Management for me!!

The Heart of a Woman
How to look after the heart you give to the world - Gill Barham
pg. 165

A true NWM business model is based on everyone doing a little and teaching others to do the same, so that it looks just like this:

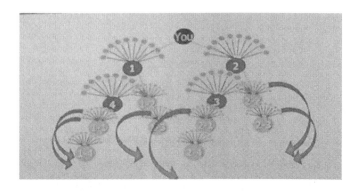

"I met Gill working in the field of nutritional health and we have formed a close partnership building a team to save 1 million lives a year focussing on heart health. Working with Gill and Synergy, I can create a passive income, create more financial security for me and my son and I love the fact that I have great mentorship and support as it can be quite isolating working for myself. Gill has many great qualities. She is always upbeat and we always have a laugh together which is so important."
Sally Varley, Acupuncturist

VIII.2
Uniqueness

There are thousands of NWM/MLM businesses out there for you to look at. My most heartfelt suggestion is that you do your due diligence on whichever company you choose. However here are a few tips that I have learned.

The Heart of a Woman
How to look after the heart you give to the world - Gill Barham
pg. 166

All great companies do 3 things

1. They solve a significant problem and fulfil a demand.

Synergy are first to market focussing on Metabolic Syndrome and the disease megatrends of the 21st century.

2. They are scalable by being relevant and compelling to a large demographic. They are:

- For everyone, regardless of age
- Measureable

3. They are unique and differentiated.

Synergy offer holistic solutions with

- Clinical evidence
- Patents
- Programmes – not just products

One of the most exciting benefits of working with Synergy is the-state-of-the-art Hughes Centre for Research and Innovation.

I am so proud to be part of their latest science based project which addresses:

Improving Metabolic Function through a Healthy Microbiome.

The Heart of a Woman
How to look after the heart you give to the world - Gill Barham

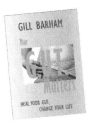

You can read much more about this in my book
Your G.U.T. Matters

*"What an amazing and professional opportunity. Truly inspirational
leaders with world beating nutritional products that leave our
competition in the supplement marketplace lagging behind. These
really are world class products grounded in science! We have
something to really be proud of, and I for one needed to grow my
belief by attending the Synergy WorldWide summit and hearing the
best leaders in this industry speak. I look forward to working with
you all, and would like to especially thank Gill, and her colleagues for
making me feel part of a great team. Onward and upward, now to
start using the new Microbiome kit."*
James Tomkies, PhysioElite Ltd

VIII.3
Compensation

If you are going to devote several years to building a residual
income, it is prudent to find a NWM company that compensates
their distributors or consultants at the highest and fairest levels. I
have seen many compensation plans, but none to beat one that
offers commission payments of 55% of company profits in bonuses;

The Heart of a Woman
How to look after the heart you give to the world - Gill Barham
pg. 168

where you are rewarded for effort that is entirely focussed on establishing a culture of generosity and service to others, where the more people you help, the more your business will grow.

Have you considered the value of developing a residual income?

You will have the opportunity to learn how you can:

Move away from *exchanging* your time for money and make money while you s*leep*
Leverage your time and effort – do something *once* but help *many* people
Increase your financial resilience by *diversifying* your income streams
Create a residual income that will grow *larger* and you grow *older*

At the very least you can create an income to cover the cost of the high quality nutrition you need to achieve Elite Health.

I support my team members by helping them to develop just a handful of clients who want better health and are drawn to natural remedies. We then help some of them or those attracted by a part-time home based business opportunity to do just the same. Synergy compensate me for my time and support in 8 different ways, including matching £ for £, or $ for $ each team member's basic commission amount each month (the unique Mega Match bonus).

The Heart of a Woman
How to look after the heart you give to the world - Gill Barham
pg. 169

Most other NWM compensation plans have a point at which payments stop as the team grows. With Synergy, this is an infinity plan, which means that there are no limits to the number of people in an individual's team.

The exciting and rewarding culture of growing a business based on great products is that an estimate of 30% of clients become team members by default as they cannot help but recommend the products when they see the results they create and the effects on lives for the better. It's a bit like getting paid for recommending a favourite restaurant or a good film (but you are rewarded for sharing).

It is hard to describe how rewarding it is to be able to offer others the opportunity to be compensated for helping to save lives every day.

**You can either
choose to be part
of the problem, or
part of the
solution.**

www.theLifestyleLeader.co.uk

LEADER

The Heart of a Woman
How to look after the heart you give to the world - Gill Barham
pg. 170

VIII.4
Compassion & Commitment

Synergy Founder, Dan Higginson leads the way in Synergy's culture of compassion. Here are just two examples of the extra ways in which Synergy offer hope, apart from the obvious passion for changing lives with the Synergy Business opportunity by giving people across 28 counties the chance to change their futures.

Team Synergy is going up against Team Nature's Sunshine Products in a friendly competition to help raise funds and awareness for the Juvenile Diabetes Research Foundation, an organization I am passionate about and determined to support. This foundation actively fights against type 1 diabetes by raising awareness, gathering new knowledge, and funding new scientific research.

Each year, about 15,000 children and 15,000 adults are diagnosed with type 1 diabetes. Currently, type 1 diabetes is an incurable disease, but, together, we have the opportunity to help make this reality a thing of the past. Synergy and NSP have elected to compete against each other in a donation battle for this wonderful foundation. I feel personally responsible to make sure Team Synergy comes out on top as I will be leading the upcoming JDRF Utah walks in Salt Lake City.

Synergy WorldWide has partnered with 5 Star Legacy Foundation to improve the lives of children and families the world over. Did you

The Heart of a Woman
How to look after the heart you give to the world - Gill Barham
pg. 171

know that nearly half of Earth's 2.2 billion children live in poverty?
Synergy and 5 Star Legacy Foundation are pouring time and
resources into improving their lives by supplying food and clothing,
increasing literacy rates, and teaching the basics of entrepreneurism
to help break the poverty cycle.

What could you do with more income?

Who could you help?

What causes would you support?

Dan Higginson decided to start his business in the most difficult
market with the highest standards and attention to detail. Synergy
started in Asia and has the highest number of distributors and
turnover in Korea and Japan than anywhere else in the world.
However, the eyes of the CEO Greg Probert have turned to Europe
where he has committed staff, money and resources to help the
European market progress. It is predicted that Synergy Europe will
be in full momentum within 12-18 months and that Synergy will
become a household name.

It is my goal to help as many people as I can to develop a second
income by helping other people battle the health mega trends of
the western world. By using their global business model, the
expertise of existing team members, the support of the European

The Heart of a Woman
How to look after the heart you give to the world - Gill Barham
pg. 172

Corporate Synergy team and the first to market, patented products, this is how I am **Building a Team to Save 1 Million Lives a Year, Every Year.**

What can you give up?

The most important aspect of building a NWM business in your "spare time", is that your "spare time" habits often get in the way. If I were to ask new members to get started by paying a tenth of their yearly income to join our team so that they could guarantee to replace or even say treble their current salary or more in 3 years, do you think they would find the pockets of time in their week to devote to developing this residual income? Do you think they would prioritise activities, change some habits for a while to achieve the lifestyle they set for themselves? Well it's likely, yes.

But if I ask them to invest the price of a new smart phone to develop the same residual income, are they likely to devote the time to it then?

No, mostly not... because it's too easy to focus on the work rather than the reward.

AND THAT'S OK IF THAT'S YOU

The Heart of a Woman
How to look after the heart you give to the world - Gill Barham
pg. 173

Our most common income streams are made by exchanging our time for money, and most people do not want to practise delayed gratification; to work now, but get paid later. However, by offering other people the chance to realise their dreams and help them to succeed so that they can have, be and do what they want, when they want, where they want, with whoever they want, we too can achieve a better lifestyle.

As a team, with regular commitment, we can help many more people around the world to live a life of Health, Happiness and Prosperity; to enjoy a true sense of Wellbeing, to be able to contribute to the world, to make a difference, leave a legacy and be the "good example".

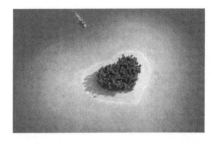

BY WORKING TOGETHER, WHO CAN WE SAVE?

The Heart of a Woman
How to look after the heart you give to the world - Gill Barham
pg. 174

VIII.5

Excellence

For me it's all about quality, quality, quality.

Most Trustworthy Companies

In 2013, Forbes Magazine published its list of **America's 100 Most Trustworthy Companies**, naming Nature's Sunshine / Synergy WorldWide under its Micro-Cap category. Being named on this list demonstrates Synergy's commitment to being "a model of openness and integrity," according to Forbes' own description.

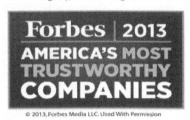

© 2013, Forbes Media LLC. Used With Permission

Synergy WorldWide was the only Direct Sales company on this list in 2013

The Synergy Advantage

When you work with a company that is cash rich and a member of NASDAQ, the benefits to the employees, distributors and clients are enhanced considerably.

This is because a company with ethics, like NSP/Synergy use their wealth to invest in people.

The Heart of a Woman
How to look after the heart you give to the world - Gill Barham
pg. 175

The scientists at the NSP (Nature's Sunshine Products) /Synergy WorldWide manufacturing plants are at the cutting edge of product development and have exceptionally sophisticated equipment available to them to perform up to 600 tests to check for quality, potency and purity on every product at every stage. The Hughes Centre has attracted eminent PhD's, herbalists, endocrinologists and pharmacognacists from all over the world because of this cutting edge research and innovation.

Chief Quality officer Lynda Hammonds describes the supplement industry as like "The Wild West without a Sherriff". 85% of supplements on the market today are "white label", in other words, made by large manufacturers and supplied to have their own labels applied. There are no requirements or regulation of these FOOD STATE supplements, so each company is responsible for their own diligence and compliance. NSP/SYNERGY take pride in their standards and compliance and are used by the FDA as the standard for nutraceutical manufacturing.

Compliant with International
Regulations

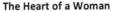

The Heart of a Woman
How to look after the heart you give to the world - Gill Barham

I was fortunate to visit the manufacturing plant in Spanish Fork, Utah with my husband in 2015. We saw for ourselves the highest levels of cleanliness, the attention to detail and precision and the quality processes and advanced equipment in the laboratories that are producing these amazing, life enhancing products.

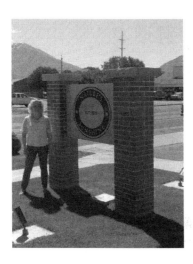

The Heart of a Woman
How to look after the heart you give to the world - Gill Barham
pg. 177

VIII.6
Simplicity

For most people who are considering joining a NWM company, the most common concern is usually "but I don't have the time".

It is true of course, that you have to dedicate time to your business, relative to what you want to achieve. The NWM industry often attracts a bad name for itself, as some company plans promise high returns for what appears to be relatively small input.

What I have found, is that, the only people that complain about NWM have either
1. Never been in the industry or
2. Started a business but didn't commit enough CONSISTENT effort for a long enough period in order to create a good foundation.
3. Didn't have a mentor or sponsor who cared about their goals and dreams more than their own.
4. The system was too complicated or there were too many products.

The most important aspect of creating a residual income is that when you move away from exchanging your time for money it takes time to build a business that delivers a consistent return. It's a bit like rolling a snowball up a hill… it's hard work until you reach the summit and then the snowball has its own momentum as it rolls

The Heart of a Woman
How to look after the heart you give to the world - Gill Barham
pg. 178

down the other side; there is almost nothing you can do to stop it at that point.

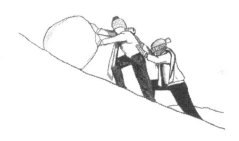

"Most distributors over-estimate the income they will make in their first 6 months of a NWM business, but will underestimate the income by year 3, IF they are persistent and consistent." **Eric Worre**

In my experience, any lack of consistency is the most common reason for failure. This usually happens when there is more focus on the work involved than **W.H.Y.** the business was attractive in the first place. Running a business like this involves stepping out of your comfort zone, so you need to work more on your mind-set than your business initially in order to overcome your own limiting beliefs, or the opinions of others.

K.I.S.S. (Keep It Simple Stupid)

The Heart of a Woman
How to look after the heart you give to the world - Gill Barham
pg. 179

There are several advantages of working with Synergy that make the time you do have available work for you. The product range is very small which means that the business model is very simple to operate and duplicate.

Nowadays with the technology available to us, we can build a business and earn while you learn by plugging in to the online training programmes and mentoring sessions available all over the world.

Who do you know with high blood pressure?

Who can you help overcome illness?

How many people do you know that are concerned about their weight?

What will you feel like when you have helped someone battle the complications of diabetes or just to sleep better or to have more energy?

What legacy can you leave working to share some natural solutions to common illness and disease?

The Heart of a Woman
How to look after the heart you give to the world - Gill Barham
pg. 180

VIII.7
Synergy

I think that SynergyWorldwide are best placed to tell you about their company's ethics and values. This is their own copy.

 # The Legacy We Create is the Legacy We Leave

Synergy WorldWide empowers people on their quests to live healthy, meaningful lives. We offer innovative business opportunities based on scientific health solutions, because we believe that when people are physically and financially able, they will make a positive difference in this world.

Solid Foundation. Proven Success.
Synergy is a Nature's Sunshine Company, internationally thriving and committed to quality, results, and integrity. Nature's Sunshine, Synergy WorldWide's publicly traded parent company, has been an industry giant for over 40 years and provides Synergy with an enormous amount of resources.

We have been named by Forbes as one of "America's 100 Most Trustworthy Companies". In fact, we were the only Direct Selling Company on the list, and one of only four companies categorized as "Pharmaceutical" to be named.

The Heart of a Woman
How to look after the heart you give to the world - Gill Barham
pg. 181

Envisioning Health & Prosperity

Dan Higginson founded Synergy in 1999 with a vision to "help people everywhere attain better health, grow more prosperous, and support communities in need." Today, that vision is becoming a reality in more than 25 markets internationally.

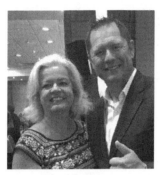

Dan Higginson

The Better You Feel, the Better You Live

As a trusted natural supplement manufacturer, we focus on helping people around the world increase health to better leave a legacy. We focus on the well-being of our customers and the reputation of our Team Members. It has been said that the greatest wealth is health, and we believe that to be true. We aim to provide the highest quality health solutions to all who seek them.

The Heart of a Woman
How to look after the heart you give to the world - Gill Barham
pg. 182

Synergy Innovation

We do our homework. At the Hughes Center for Research and Innovation, Synergy's state-of- the-art clinic and laboratory space, our Medical & Scientific Advisory Board and their staff work continuously to develop real health solutions for a world in need.

Synergy Innovation (2)

The Synergy Medical & Scientific Advisory Board is composed of doctors, scientists, and leaders in the field of health and nutrition. Dr. Matthew Tripp is our company's Chief Scientific Officer and serves as the head of this Advisory Board. As a doctor of physiology, microbial genetics, and microbiology with more than 100 patents under his name, Dr. Tripp has dedicated his extensive career to managing the discovery, development, safety, and clinical validation of medical foods and nutraceuticals.

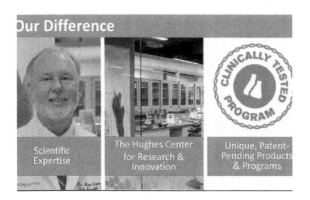

The Heart of a Woman
How to look after the heart you give to the world - Gill Barham

"My passion is making a difference in the world. You might call it a personal mission, if you will. It's not religion based, it's just seeing a great level of chronic illness in the world and asking, 'How can I make a difference?' and 'How can we work together?"

Dr Matt Tripp

The Heart of a Woman
How to look after the heart you give to the world - Gill Barham
pg. 184

Synergy Manufacturing.

At Synergy, we formulate and proudly create the products that are improving lives around the world. Our manufacturing facility is NSF certified and is recognized for excellence in manufacturing practices. We refuse to leave the quality of our products in the hands of anyone else.

Synergy Quality Assurance.

We ensure quality from start to finish. The Synergy Quality Assurance department performs thorough audits around the world at the source of our ingredients. Upon arrival, those ingredients are tested to confirm identity, safety, and potency. Additionally, every lot we manufacture goes through additional testing. This multi-million Dollar annual investment in quality ensures a finished product you can count on.

Synergy's premiere health enhancement product is ProArgi-9+.

2016 US Physicians' Desk Reference
ProArgi-9+ is the only L-Arginine supplement in the book

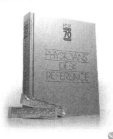

"ProArgi-9+ is the highest quality L-Arginine supplement in the world. This proprietary formulation combines the powerful cardiovascular benefits of L-Arginine with a variety of superior heart health ingredients to give your cardiovascular system optimum support."

The Heart of a Woman
How to look after the heart you give to the world - Gill Barham

TRUSTED.

For decades, we have worked to earn our reputation and live by our mission statement. From entrepreneurs and business professionals, to world-class athletes from around the world, millions of people have put Synergy to the test. Our products and our company are changing lives every day.

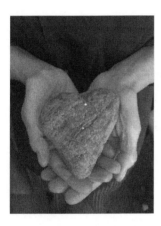

Your future is in your own hands.

The Heart of a Woman
How to look after the heart you give to the world - Gill Barham
pg. 186

CHAPTER VIII

Purpose

One of the biggest and most important messages that I have heard time and again from the many mentors and successful entrepreneurs that I am fortunate to spend time with, is that to feel fulfilled in life, you need to work out what you are passionate about so that you can make it your life's purpose. Or if you want to live a healthier life, then taking time to examine the impact of that is a vital step towards achieving success.

What I have found, is that the women whom I admire, live their lives with a sense of purpose, make a contribution with their skills and talents, are happy and fulfilled, are comfortable with expressing their emotions, stand up for what they believe in and have the ability to bring out the best in others. I am wondering what attributes you like about the women you love?

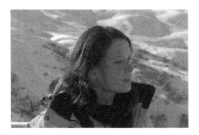

The Heart of a Woman
How to look after the heart you give to the world - Gill Barham

A useful exercise for you to do:

1. Who do you admire in your family?

WHY?

2. Who do you admire in your circle of friends?

WHY?

3. Who do you admire from history or the media?

WHY?

4. Do any of these people have any of these attributes?

- a good sense of themselves
- confidence
- passion and purpose
- a sense of humour
- a happy disposition
- generosity
- leadership
- grace
- talent
- a good work ethic
- a healthy body/mindset
- a caring attitude
- empathy
- drive

The Heart of a Woman
How to look after the heart you give to the world - Gill Barham
pg. 188

- honesty
- the ability to laugh at themselves
- acceptance that life has ups and downs

.... what else?

Are there any common traits or attributes amongst them all?

The chances are that you will be drawn to the very things that you value, aspire to and that you already possess, even if you don't realise it yet.

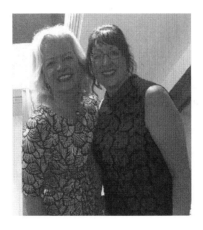

Me with Cheryl

The Heart of a Woman
How to look after the heart you give to the world - Gill Barham
pg. 189

I believe that you have one person (me) and at least one more, or even lots of other people that admire YOU too. You may not currently feel like you are achieving your dreams, living life to the full, or just being you, but **The Rapid Realignment Process™** is going to help you to do just that.

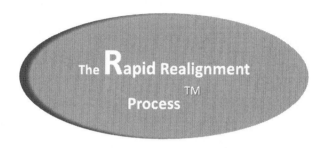

VII.1 It's all about finding your W.H.Y.

This book would not have happened were it not for the friendship, leadership and mentorship of the amazing Cheryl Chapman, or Queen C, as I call her.

With her "partner in crime", Marion Bevington, who is equally amazing by the way, her specialty is helping you find your WHY. As I have benefitted from their wisdom, I cannot help but share a little of the work that has been a catalyst for growth and prosperity for me and my fellow mentees.

The Heart of a Woman
How to look after the heart you give to the world - Gill Barham
pg. 190

"When you find something that just feels right –it will encourage you, and it will give you energy and motivation. It helps you to work in harmony with your brain and your body, and that is why knowing your WHY is crucial for you."

"Find Your Why: To become Frickin' Awesome" by Cheryl Chapman

The Heart of a Woman
How to look after the heart you give to the world - Gill Barham
pg. 191

However, it was many, many years ago that I discovered for myself that in order to have a sense of wellbeing, to be happy and fulfilled, to feel valued and valuable, it is a really good idea to take a look at W.H.Y. you are here, what you want to leave as a legacy and who you want to influence. In other words, finding your PURPOSE.

Once you find your purpose, your life will take on a new meaning and so will your sense of wellbeing.

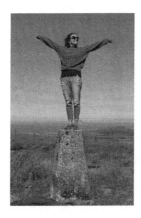

It's all about passion!!

Of all the entrepreneurs I have worked with, met and studied, they all have the same thing in common: they have either
- made a business out of something they are passionate about OR
- they have become passionate about a business or "Cause" they have been introduced to.

The Heart of a Woman
How to look after the heart you give to the world - Gill Barham
pg. 192

"Passion pushes you to complete your dreams.
Purpose is a happy place where you are in balance and fulfilled."
Jayne Bernard

The Heart of a Woman
How to look after the heart you give to the world - Gill Barham
pg. 193

The 3 parts of **The Rapid Realignment Process™** will help you to start the process to finding your **W.H.Y.** as we work together through each part:

The
Wellbeing Wheel™
The
Happy Habit Blueprint™
And
Your Self-Talk Tracker™

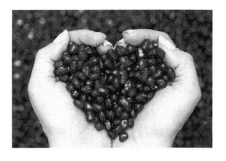

The Heart of a Woman
How to look after the heart you give to the world - Gill Barham
pg. 194

VII.2 Let's start with The **W**ellbeing Wheel™

The Wellbeing Wheel™

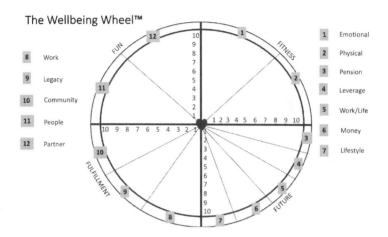

8	Work		1	Emotional
9	Legacy		2	Physical
10	Community		3	Pension
11	People		4	Leverage
12	Partner		5	Work/Life
			6	Money
			7	Lifestyle

This is a critical exercise to do whatever you had in your mind when you decided to read this book.

As part of the online programme we look at four areas of your life in more detail. At the end of the book there is a link to a pdf version of this exercise for you to print off, in which case you will need some paper, a pen and some quiet time alone to complete this successfully.

Please look at each section in turn. Firstly, make some notes about how you feel about each of these areas. I have posed a few questions for each to get you thinking.

The Heart of a Woman
How to look after the heart you give to the world - Gill Barham
pg. 195

Fitness

1. Emotional health – e.g. are you happy, contented, depressed, sad, frustrated. Do you have some "me" time scheduled in? What is your favourite way to relax and revive and do you do this regularly enough? Do you spend time and money on any personal development programmes and regular health or beauty treatments?

2. Physical health – e.g. do you feel as physically fit as you would like? Are you at your ideal weight? Do you have any health issues?

Future

3. Pension/security - are you confident about your financial resilience? Is your future secure enough not to have to rely on a pension?

4. Leverage - Do you have a plan B? Do you have a way to create a residual income? What would happen to your income if you were unable to work for any reason? Do you lie awake worrying about money?

5. Work/life balance – are you happy with the amount of time you have to spend with loved ones, are you working more hours than you would like?

The Heart of a Woman
How to look after the heart you give to the world - Gill Barham
pg. 196

6. Money/debt - do you owe money? Do you have savings? Do you pay into a pension or have investments?

7. Lifestyle – are you living the life that you imagined for yourself or have you cut your cloth and reduced your expectations of what you want or maybe what you deserve?

Ask yourself questions like: "where do I see myself in 5, 10, 20 years?", "what do I want in my life" and "what will my life be like?".

Fulfillment

8. Job/business – is this making you happy? Do you work with like-minded souls who appreciate and respect you? Do you live for your days off? Are you a stay at home Mum feeling bored or frustrated, (even though you love being a parent)? Are you looking for a new challenge? Are you using your skills or just working to make money?

*These are some of the most common comments I see when we do this exercise in The **Your Heart Matters™** Programme:*

I feel busy, but not fulfilled" or "I'm not sure where I'm heading any more", "I feel like I have lost sight of my dreams", "I used to know what I wanted ... but I don't know now."

9. Leaving your legacy – what do you want people to say about you when you die? Will you have left your mark? Who are you helping and influencing now?

The Heart of a Woman
How to look after the heart you give to the world - Gill Barham
pg. 197

"With every word we utter, with every action we take, we know our kids are watching us" Michelle Obama

10. Community collaboration / cooperation – are you part of any groups or clubs, past times or self-improvement associations? Do you contribute to any good causes? Are you able to find ways to feel valued and valuable?

You could ask yourself questions like: "what do I really want to have achieved?" "what do I want to feel proud of?", "what have I always wanted to do?"

Fun and recreation

11. Friends and family – Do you spend enough or too much time with the people you love? Do they nourish you? Is your friendship an equal one?

12. Relationships – how happy are you with your partner or are you happy to be single?

Now….. In the Your H.E.A.R.T. Matters ™ programme I ask my clients to give each of these sections a score and chart these scores onto

The Heart of a Woman
How to look after the heart you give to the world - Gill Barham
pg. 198

The Wellbeing Wheel™ filling in each triangle so that it will look a little like this one. Complete each section where 10 is bad and 1 is fab.

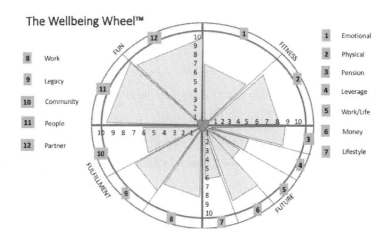

This gives a visual image of where they most need to focus their attention.

In the example above, this lady was struggling mostly with her relationships and having fun. She was also able to identfy that she needed to address some issues around her physical health, her current financial situation. She also recognised that she had a poor sense of purpose and what her legacy will look like.

The Heart of a Woman
How to look after the heart you give to the world - Gill Barham
pg. 199

Every picture tells a story

Do you remember the exercise we did in Chapter III**?** What does your ideal day look like?

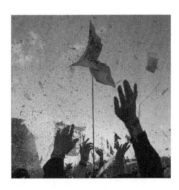

How would you like your life to be?

Look again at the notes you made from that exercise. Close your eyes and imagine how you will feel when you achieve this.

How does that day compare to the exercise you have just completed? Can you see now where the main focus of your attention should or could be?

The Heart of a Woman
How to look after the heart you give to the world - Gill Barham
pg. 200

I would like to share with you my 50 top tips to help you achieve a life of Wellbeing - Optimum Health, Wealth and Happiness.

We have covered some aspects already, but here we have a quick guide all in one place.

Self-Care

1. **Drink at least 8 glasses of water a day** and cut out the caffeine! Our bodies are composed of 60-70% water and you need to drink enough to keep your bodily joints working, maintain energy and perform at your peak. If you are thirsty, you are already dehydrated.
2. **Try to move more regularly**: Make time to do some sort of physical activity, whether it's a brisk walk, a Lifestyle Pilates™ online session, or a swim or fitness session. You know your body will thank you for it. If you are desk bound, make sure you get up and about every hour.
3. **Learn about good nutrition**: Sort through the myths surrounding low fat, low carb, fad diets and packaged 'health food' products.
4. **Try to eat whole foods and organic produce**: The less processed the better; higher in nutrients, lower in toxins, better for the earth and pure - free from chemicals and genetic modification...

The Heart of a Woman
How to look after the heart you give to the world - Gill Barham
pg. 201

5. **Plan your meals** a week ahead: This avoids unnecessary take-aways and reduces the cost of waste. Having a menu plan will also help you maintain your new healthy eating habits.
6. **Take a good quality multivitamin** and mineral supplement: It can be tough trying to achieve your daily recommended 7 servings of fresh fruits and vegetables. When you consider the nutrition that's lost through the modern farming, packaging and transportation processes, it makes sense to take a good quality supplement and support your health.
7. **Ditch the bad habits**: Smoking, excessive alcohol intake and drugs are damaging for the body, sometimes ruining relationships as well as ending lives. (Not you obviously)
8. **Maintain your ideal weight**: Study the health advice in The **Your H.E.A.R.T. Matters™** Programme to learn how to do this with ease.
9. **Relax**: Stress is the biggest epidemic in the western world and a major contributing factor to many illnesses and disease.
10. **Sleep more**: In order to repair and rejuvenate, make sure that you are getting enough sleep every night so you can take on each day full of vitality. Have a night time routine, turn off laptops, tablets and phones and if you wake up regularly in the small hours, try eating a little before bedtime. (A couple of Oatcakes are good.)
11. **Spend time in nature**: Being outdoors in nature for just 20 minutes can boost your vitality; can instantly increase your sense of wellbeing and ward off feelings of exhaustion. You will also get some essential vitamin D3. (You should DEFINITELY be supplementing with this in the autumn and winter months as well)
12. **Set yourself a physical challenge** whether big or small. Try walking more, set a physical challenge, overcome a fear to

prove to yourself that anything is possible which will improve your confidence and sense of achievement.

13. **Look into natural and alternative therapies**: Understand that everything put into your body will create a chemical reaction. Prescribed and 'over the counter' medications can have potentially deadly side-effects.

14. **Love the body you've got** and familiarise yourself with what's normal for you and what's not. With all its perfect imperfections, it's all you've got so make sure you cherish it!

Self-Growth

15. **Believe in yourself** no matter what you're up against: "Whether you think you can or you think you can't, you're right" - HENRY FORD

16. **Tell yourself the right story**: Often, the only thing holding you back is the story you tell yourself. Get a new story and start living.

17. **Have an Attitude of Gratitude**: Be grateful for what you have; look around and be in the moment. Find five things and say it out loud.

18. **Have confidence to be the real woman** that you are. Ask yourself if you are acting, reacting and interacting in a way that matches the unique sense of your **feminine self**.

19. **Read some inspiring motivational books or listen to podcasts** relevant to the areas of your life that you want to improve.

20. **Set your alarm** 15 minutes earlier than normal so you can start your day less rushed and more in control.

The Heart of a Woman
How to look after the heart you give to the world - Gill Barham
pg. 203

Self-Improvement

21. **Tell someone that you love them,** more regularly and in a variety of ways!

22. **Meditate**: this will help you feel more alive, energised and reduce stress and anxiety; it's a fantastic way to spend a few minutes of calm mindfulness every day to really be in the moment. I use "My Headspace", an online, easy to use and inexpensive led meditation programme.

23. **Regularly visit all the good things about you**: Remember, you are your own unique being. Take time to appreciate how amazing you already are. If you are not feeling confident about this, ask your friends what they think are your best qualities.

24. **Reward your achievements**: Recognise every milestone that you pass and celebrate the small successes. Buy yourself a small treat or take time for some "me time" with a walk, a good book, film, or a hair or beauty treatment.

25. **Surround yourself with people who lift you up** not drag you down: "You are the average of the five people you spend the most time with". Make sure they're the people who emulate what you want to be known for.

26. **Take stock and reassess the relationships** in your life: Choose who you associate with and be prepared to set up boundaries with any negative influences in your life, this includes the people you spend time with on your TV or radio!

27. **Place your favourite inspirational quotes** into frames and put them in prominent places. Make a picture vision board and hang it in a prominent place or make one to use as a **screen saver**.

28. **Get into the habit** of bringing **fresh flowers** inside.

The Heart of a Woman
How to look after the heart you give to the world - Gill Barham
pg. 204

29. **DE clutter**. DE clutter. DE clutter: A clear and organised environment encourages a clear and organised life.
30. **Hold a table top sale** or give unwanted items to charity. Let go of possessions that no longer fulfil a purpose for you or bring joy to your life.
31. **Put your special occasion** and beautiful possessions on display: And use them!
32. **Put on some music** that gets you grooving: Think of your life as needing a sound track and you have the ability to affect the story of your life through music. Just make sure that you pick positive and inspiring tunes as listening to depressing songs can have the opposite effect, encouraging you to wallow in self-pity.
33. **Create a photo album** of favourite happy memories and take the time to go through it often.
34. **Work with a MUST list. Not a to-do list.** A 'must' list should only have 3-5 tasks that must get done today and should attempt to be achieved no matter what. Long lists destroy motivation and while they're necessary to stay organised, they shouldn't be your go-to visual for how to tackle the day. Top Tip: Use a post-it pad, so that you can tear off each task as you go!

Self-Awareness

35. **Slow down**: When you slow down the pace of life, you create space to do what truly inspires you.

The Heart of a Woman
How to look after the heart you give to the world - Gill Barham
pg. 205

36. **Embrace your uniqueness**: Realise that there is only one you for a reason - that you have something worthwhile to contribute to the world in your own special way.

37. **Create affirmations** that resonate with you: Positive phrases that you repeat out loud to yourself reprogram your brain to seek out opportunities and transform into truth. I use Subliminal360, a visual and audio programme available for laptops (but not macs).

38. **Focus on fun**: Too often we get caught up in the detail and demands of the day-to-day. Life is here to be enjoyed. If money were not an issue, what would you be spending your time doing?

39. **Get over your fears and doubts**: There'll never be the perfect time to get started. You can achieve anything. So start today!

40. **Delegate and outsource** where you can to free up time to focus on your passion and what really inspires you. Outsourcing mundane tasks such as ironing, cleaning, even hiring a virtual assistant can free up precious time in your everyday life.

41. **Take up studying** in the areas that most inspire you: Education is a powerful tool and we all have a need to grow. You're never too old to start and you may never be old enough to stop.

42. **Give back**: Find a cause that's important to you and support it.

43. **Develop a bucket list**: Every person has limited time on this planet with so much to do and see. It's important to define what's most important for you to experience in this life.

44. **Take a different route to work**: It's a great feeling to occasionally step outside of your comfort zone and see the world from a different perspective.

45. **Don't be afraid to change direction**: You will be pleasantly surprised at how easy it is when you make the decision to move

The Heart of a Woman
How to look after the heart you give to the world - Gill Barham
pg. 206

away from what is making you unhappy or frustrated. All the better if you can find someone to help you.

46. **Stop multi-tasking everything in your life.** Sometimes multi-tasking is necessary and a useful tool but used too often and in areas where a single focus would achieve more can end up being counter-productive. More on this later.

47. **Develop some goals are turn them into a VISION**... imagine what you see, hear, feel and say when you have successfully achieved it. Write it down, look at it and speak this out loud every day.

48. **Make a deliberate effort NOT to fill up your calendar.** Leave space for creativity, for spontaneity and for some "me time".

49. **Get up early now-and-then to watch the sunrise**: Because every new day is a new opportunity, a new experience and a chance to live life exactly as you desire.

50. **Keep up with friends**: call or meet-up regularly with those special ladies in your life for a laugh and a gossip!

Have a go at a selection of these at a time, and notice how you feel.

The Heart of a Woman
How to look after the heart you give to the world - Gill Barham
pg. 207

VII.4 Your Self-Talk Tracker™

The more frequently and thoroughly you work on how you want to live in the world, the more opportunity you will have to create that life for yourself. By the way, I was very skeptical when I first started to practice visualisation and self-talk techniques, but what I found is that you get most of what you think most about!!

This is your opportunity to get familiar with what you say when you talk to yourself!
A few common examples:
- I can't lose weight
- I'll never be successful in business
- I am never going to find the right partner
- I have heart disease/cancer in my family, so I expect it will get me too in the end.
- I'll never be able do that
- Nobody will want to hear what I think
- I don't think that person/people like me

What is interesting, is that all of these insecurities are based on 3 basic lies

1. I'm not good enough
2. I can't cope, it's all too much
3. I'm unlovable, I am not worthy

Some, if not all of these limiting beliefs stem from your earliest days as a young child and are often picked up from your parents. It's a bit like the snake phobia, (which I have now overcome), that came from

The Heart of a Woman
How to look after the heart you give to the world - Gill Barham
pg. 208

my mother. You see your mind is like a mad dog on a lead! It is pulling you around and confusing you all the time.

Why would it do that, you may wonder?

The job of the mind is to keep you safe – it likes the familiar, it is telling you "better the devil you know." That's why we get stuck in life; just like your suitcase on the carousel at the airport going round and round until you take action to pull it off. We feel safe with what we already know. However:

Your freedom actually lies in the unknown and everything you need is already inside of you.

www.theLifestyleLeader.co.uk

You can change your self-talk and your vision for your future:
- It's easy for me to lose weight and keep it off
- I am making the difference I want to make because my business is growing everyday
- I always find the right people to spend time with, and my soulmate is just around the corner
- I am enjoying looking after myself, so that I will live a healthy and happy life.
- I am loved, I am worthy, I am everything I need to be and more

The Heart of a Woman
How to look after the heart you give to the world - Gill Barham

What is your vision for your future?

Having, or developing a vision does not mean you are unhappy with your life right now, and it does not mean you cannot live in the moment, embracing life in the here and now.

A vision is not an objective or goal. It does not need to be "specific, measurable, achievable, realistic, time-related". (you know about SMART goals right?) It may never be reported against, or ticked off. In fact, it may well continue to develop over time, and continue to be slightly elusive, just there on the horizon.

However, it will help you to form your **Intentions.**

A vision can broaden your horizons and create new challenges for yourself. It will help you to feel excited about the future; make you feel you want to take action towards it, and will even help you to expand your comfort zone, and take more risks. Keeping your vision in mind through the inevitable challenges of working towards your new intentions, can also really help maintain commitment levels and enable you to overcome hurdles.

So now write down the ONE THING that you would like to change first.....and then what that change or improvement would do to positively influence the other areas of your life at present.

For example: I would like to work with people more like me, so my one intention for the next six weeks is to find another job or business that will make me feel more confident and fulfilled.

The Heart of a Woman
How to look after the heart you give to the world - Gill Barham
pg. 210

This is likely to be the one thing that you will set as your intention to work on as part of The **Your H.E.A.R.T. Matters™** Programme.

Now you need to verbalise that every day, put it in front of you in very way you can think of.

Once you have a clear intention about what you want to achieve this will help you to take appropriate action and keep you on track. With our very busy lives, perhaps it is all too easy to get distracted or maybe you even suffer from procrastination? That is why the six online weekly mentorship programme for six to ten ladies works well, especially for women, as together we achieve more when we help and support each other.

Having a community of ladies all on a similar path, even with very different intentions, has such an impact on the results, that I invite the ladies on The **Your H.E.A.R.T. Matters™** Programme into our exclusive Facebook group for extra support, **The Homeplace**, because "home is where the heart is".

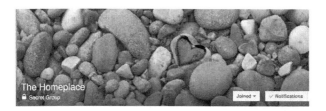

So now that we have explored your **W.H.Y.**

The Heart of a Woman
How to look after the heart you give to the world - Gill Barham
pg. 211

LET'S GET YOU IN ACTION

Once you decide on the ONE intention that you want to concentrate on, as part of The **Your H.E.A.R.T. Matters**™ Programme, we can start to work together to achieve your aim.

In my experience, here are few things that get in our way when we set a new intention:

- Fear of failure
- Procrastination
- Feeling unworthy
- Feeling that you are not good enough
- Worried about being judged or criticised
- Fear of success
- Fear of change
- Peer pressure to stay the same
- Negative self-talk
- Feeling that you won't cope

However, there are ways that you can overcome these emotions and feelings that have the potential to hold you back, and once learned, can be used for any subsequent goals, dreams and intentions that you set yourself for the future.

Remember I said I overcame my phobia of snakes? Well I had help from the lovely Marion. She has a variety of approaches to facilitate change, which is what we need to do here to create some good habits and get you moving towards your dreams.

The Heart of a Woman
How to look after the heart you give to the world - Gill Barham
pg. 212

"You've got to change the emotion in order to change feeling – then the thinking, then the behavior."

Marion Bevington

The Heart of a Woman
How to look after the heart you give to the world - Gill Barham
pg. 213

Here are some more details on just a selection of the 50 Fulfillment tips;

Secret no 1

Support and collaboration is key. Being part of a community of like-minded people, receiving praise, where deserved and encouragement, when needed. This is what my clients appreciate most with the **Your H.E.A.R.T. Matters™** Community.

"We are the average of the five people we spend the most time with" Jim Rohn

The Heart of a Woman
How to look after the heart you give to the world - Gill Barham
pg. 214

Secret no 2

What helps with achieving your intention is to anchor it in some way. This can be in any form you find useful - a list, an object, a short phrase, a collage or vision board, a diagram, a reminder on your fridge, a letter to yourself perhaps?

Having an attitude of gratitude

Here is just one example of something you may like to try.

At the end of each day do you berate yourself for things that didn't go to plan, mistakes you made and things you missed? Or do you remember all of the mini wins of the day?

Do you go to sleep hearing the negative comments, daily news stories or media sound bites in your head? Or do you remember all the little kind gestures and moments of love or friendship you experienced during the day?

Happiness is usually just a small step away from most people but unfortunately (mainly because of our overloaded information age) it is too easy to focus on the tragedies, the upsets and troubles of the world and our place in it. We may also be trapped into worrying about the opinions others may have of us, when really they are just keeping their heads above water too!

Here's two quick ways to focus on what's going well:

The Heart of a Woman
How to look after the heart you give to the world - Gill Barham
pg. 215

1. Write down 5 mini wins every night (no matter how small).

Do every night for 1 year and you will have recorded 1825 wins!

And do you remember tip no 17?

2. Write down 5 things you are grateful for.

Today I am grateful for...................
Today I am grateful for...................
Today I am grateful for...................
Today I am grateful for...................
Today I am grateful for...................

Putting these into practice will build your self-esteem, help you to focus on what's really important in your life and ultimately, increase your sense of wellbeing.

Power up

What I have discovered by working with Cheryl and Marion, is that, whilst vision boards may work for some people, it is even better to create a "sensory" board. This 3D version is more powerful and allows for the vision of your future to grow as your horizons expand. Instead of random pictures cut out of magazines, which is what I used to do, it is much more impactful to personalise your images, adding sounds and smells, updates, awards and achievements. Building outwards on top of older posts. You get the picture?

The Heart of a Woman
How to look after the heart you give to the world - Gill Barham
pg. 216

Secret no 3

But there is one important thing that achieves the best results when setting your intention. It is about having some accountability. That is why slimming groups work, in the short term at least; why we achieve stuff at school, or as an employee, in sport, particularly as part of a team, and how we succeed in our relationships.

And we either
1. respond by moving towards something we want, or
2. away from something we don't want.

Which one motivates you the most?

In the **Your H.E.A.R.T. Matters™** Programme we work that out to help you achieve your intention.

What just happened?

This is exciting. Once you focus on your intention, this is what you will find. You will naturally filter out the people, chores, events, past-times; any and all distractions that are taking you away from the task in hand. This allows you to evaluate your daily decisions, become more organised, feel accomplished and keep on track for the time period you have set yourself.

By setting an intention, rather than a goal, (where you often feel a failure if you don't make the deadline) this affords a more open approach so that you can be more aware of other opportunities that fit in with your intention and perhaps even enhance it. When I set my first intention, I cannot tell you how doors started opening for

The Heart of a Woman
How to look after the heart you give to the world - Gill Barham
pg. 217

me and people who came into my life that have been so important to my success and sense of fulfillment. Many of these people have been a great help too in keeping me on track whilst writing this book.

Secret No 4

Multitask – me?

As women we are told that we very good at multitasking and indeed I would consider that I'm pretty good at it myself. But I thought now would be a good time to throw in my thoughts on this.

There is a place for multitasking if, like me, you have brought up children. I know that you can do the washing-up, answer the phone, feed a child, sort out the mess that the dog has made, put away the shopping - you get the idea - all without really thinking about it.

However, in business I have realised that it may not be such a good thing. If you work in an office so if you're like me and you work from home, does multitasking have a place?

Especially whilst writing this book, my experience has been pretty much a resounding NO! I have found that when I try to do more than one thing at a time, it will take much longer to do.

Let me explain what I mean. If you are going to compose an email, for example, it may take you 15 minutes. However, how easy is it to become distracted by the phone, your mobile, checking your social media, your emails, or whatever? Perhaps you have somebody else

The Heart of a Woman
How to look after the heart you give to the world - Gill Barham
pg. 218

in the house or in your place of work who interrupts you or your thought processes? Studies have shown that it will take you at least three times as long to compose that email because every time you go back to it, you are almost going to have to start where you left off; to familiarise yourself with the subject, the tone, the message you want to put across and somehow you lose the "flow" of your message. So what works for me, to save time and to achieve the best results, is to restrict myself to doing one thing at a time. So although I CAN multitask, I DON'T multitask, especially with something that is important.

So once you have set your intention, when you are approached by someone to do something that is not relevant or would slow your progress down, you are much more empowered to stick to your guns and focus on your own needs. This way of working towards your intention brings advantages that you may not expect such as; less stress in your daily life, inner peace, confidence, and a sense of control and fulfilment. It's all about the journey. You will learn to trust your gut feelings and become more selfish, I mean in a good way! So whether you want to lose weight, reverse ageing and disease, prevent illness, get fitter, learn to love yourself, secure your financial future, make new friends, improve your relationships, find a new purpose, make a speech, prepare a presentation or write a book (!!), you will achieve more when you find your **W.H.Y.**

The Heart of a Woman
How to look after the heart you give to the world - Gill Barham
pg. 219

"Before you agree to do anything that might add even the smallest amount of stress to your life, ask yourself: what is my truest intention? Give yourself time to let a "yes" resound within you. When it is right, I guarantee that your entire body will feel it."
Oprah Winfrey

The Heart of a Woman
How to look after the heart you give to the world - Gill Barham
pg. 220

CHAPTER IX

How can I support you?

Congratulations, you have reached the end of this book. How do you feel? Are you feeling positive, or have you had some time to reflect on what you may need to change to be able to see more, be more and do more in the future? I hope you have picked up some tips for healthy living, some inspiration to put yourself and your needs first as a woman and to think about how you influence others by your actions.

After all: **Actions Speak Louder Than Words.**

Here are the links to the WELLNESS QUESTIONNAIRE and the WELLBEING WHEEL for you to download. You can email me for a copy of either document and If you would like my help to complete either of these or if you have any questions, then get in touch on Gill@theLifestyleLeader.co.uk

I would love to connect with you in person. Please do find me on these social media platforms

FACEBOOK   TWITTER   LINKEDIN   YOUTUBE

And if you could post a photo of yourself with this book, that would be fantastic!
The Heart of a Woman
How to look after the heart you give to the world - Gill Barham

Bonus

I have uploaded one of the episodes of The Miracle Molecule show link here:
RADIO W.O.R.K.S. WORLD
6 facts and myths about cholesterol and statins

You can get the details of how you can work with me directly from my website: www.theLifestyleLeader.co.uk

And finally, I want to thank you from my "HEART" for reading and sharing this book and as an extra bonus, I invite you to apply for a place on my signature programme **Your H.E.A.R.T. Matters™** and receive a special discount of £100, just quote: PURE 21 as the promotional code.

The Heart of a Woman
How to look after the heart you give to the world - Gill Barham
pg. 222

Printed in Poland
by Amazon Fulfillment
Poland Sp. z o.o., Wrocław